D0651446

# The Last Chance Diet

*Dr. Linn's Protein-Sparing Fast Program*

# THE LAST

*Lyle Stuart, Inc.*  *Secaucus, N. J.*

# CHANCE DIET

*—when everything else has failed*

*by* DR. ROBERT LINN
*with* SANDRA LEE STUART

First printing, July 1976
Second printing, August 1976

Copyright © 1976 by Robert Linn and Sandra Lee Stuart

All rights reserved, including the right to quote from
or reproduce this book or any parts thereof in any form
in any part of the world.

Queries regarding rights and permissions should be addressed
to: Lyle Stuart, 120 Enterprise Avenue, Secaucus, N.J. 07094.

Published simultaneously in Canada by George J. McLeod Limited,
73 Bathurst St., Toronto, Ont.

Manufactured in the United States of America

LIBRARY OF CONGRESS CATALOGING IN PUBLICATION DATA

Linn, Robert, 1933-
    The last chance diet.

    Bibliography:  p. 245
    1.  Reducing diets.  2.  Fasting.  3.  High-protein
diet.  I.  Stuart, Sandra Lee, joint author.  II.  Title.
RM222.2.L52          613.2'5          76-19087
ISBN 0-8184-0239-3

To  Dianne

# Acknowledgments

A book is very seldom the product of one person. Others, through encouragement and advice contribute to making something work. My effort here is no exception. But how do you really thank someone like my associates in Pennsylvania and New York, Dr. Stephen Moses and Dr. Howard Shapiro? Or my Beverly Hills associate, Dr. Paul Lessler? Or Willard Krehl, M.D., Ph.D. and Alvin Goldfarb, M.D., for their ever-helpful criticisms and suggestions? I must also try to thank Maxene Kaizen, Doris Mallon, Elizabeth Faber and the rest of my invaluable staff for the help they've given. Above all, thanks to my collaborator, Sandra Lee Stuart.

And then, of course, there are many other friends and colleagues who in one way or another made this book possible. To all, perhaps, the best way to put it is simply, "Thank you."

# Contents

# Prologue to My Fellow Physicians

Dear Colleague:

Totally frustrating and often appalling!

We all have the overweight patient who dabbles on his own with one diet after another. He tortures his body by piling up those injurious extra pounds and then tortures it more by wrenching them off through one exotic and dubious means after another.

And then, on goes the weight again, and the obese patient is more so than ever.

Through it all, the patient usually neglects even the most basic principles of sound medicine and sensible health practices.

He or she is a do-it-yourselfer. As the doctor, you can only hope that no permanent damage is done.

Frustrating. The obese patient gets heavier.

Appalling. The potential harm to overweight fad dieters is, as we all know, enormous.

Be prepared for some of your patients to approach you about this protein-sparing fast program. I have counseled them to go to you. This fast cannot and should not be done without your supervision.

This could be their "last-chance" diet.

It will work.

But most important, it is safe.

Although at first glance this fasting program might seem extreme, remember, your patients are desperately in need of losing weight. They have probably tried everything else. If their dieting history hasn't been an out-and-out failure, whatever weight they did manage to take off went right back on again. They have never been able to get *enough* weight off.

This program does work—and I can show you why. I have included a bibliography on this program for your use. Reserve judgment on this type of fast until you've looked over the detailed research and studies supporting it. If you have any trouble obtaining the journals and articles listed, send a request on your professional letterhead, and I will be more than happy to forward them to you.

This program allows your patients to reach a "normal" weight rapidly. There is immediate gratification. No waiting six months, a year or two years—a long time to keep someone highly motivated—for results to show. With the continuous positive reinforcement of rapid reduction, it is much easier for the fat patient to stay with the program.

I have used these techniques on some 1800 patients over the last two years.

The protein-sparing fast is grounded on tested medical and scientific findings. The underlying concept of this type of fast began to be developed in 1967 by George Cahill, Jr., M.D., a professor of medicine at Harvard University and head of the Joslin Diabetes Foundation. It was he who studied and reported the physiology of the ketone bodies produced in fasting. It was George Blackburn, M.D., director of Nutritional Support Services at the New England Deaconess Hospital and an assistant professor of surgery at the Harvard Medical School, who earned his Ph.D. from M.I.T. developing the concept of the protein-sparing fast itself.

Needless to say, there were pioneers in the field. The modified fasting program is an evolutionary derived physiological response which was first recognized by F. M. Allen prior to the discovery of insulin.

Victor Vertes, M.D., Director of Medicine at Mt. Sinai Hospital of Cleveland and Professor of Medicine at Case Western Reserve University has done considerable work in the field of supplementary fasting of ambulatory patients.

Peter Lindner, M.D., F.I.C.A., F.R.S.H. has provided medicine with valuable reports on his clinical investigative work with supplemented outpatient fasting.

Weight reduction is but a part of the program. Integral and vital to it is the behavioral modification follow-up. This is a multi-phasic approach. Weight reduction without application of the behaviorial modification is worthless. For much of the behavior modification knowledge and techniques I am indebted to Henry A. Jordon, M.D. Associate Professor of Psychiatry, and Leonard S. Levitz, Ph.D., Assistant Professor of Psychology in the Department of Psychiatry—both at the University of Pennsylvania School of Medicine.

This book is primarily for your patient. To give him or her hope and enough self-motivation to go to you and stick with it.

DR. ROBERT LINN

*Broomall, Pa.*
July, 1976

# To the Reader

Fat.
Obese.
Overweight.
Tubby.
Portly.
Corpulent.
Rotund.
Call yourself anything you want. You know what you are.

It bothers you. It depresses you. And it should frighten you. You've been warned, time and time again, what that oppressive extra burden could mean to your health —high blood pressure, heart attack, diabetes . . . early death. . . . If your fat doesn't shorten your life, it surely makes it less rewarding, exciting, worth living. You are sentenced to death row in a prison of your own adipose tissue.

You've tried to escape by using one diet, one regimen, after another.

One month you kept Florida prosperous with all the grapefruits you bought.

Another month it was the alchemic pill you got by sending $5.95 through the mail. "Guaranteed to turn ugly fat into sensuous sinew."

You tried Stillman, Atkins, Rubin, the Air Force.

You counted calories. Computed carbohydrates. Calculated carbo-cals.

You drank enough water to float Christina Onassis' newest supertanker.

In desperation, you may have stopped eating altogether.

What did it get you? The pointer still zooms up to a depressingly high number every time you muster enough courage to step on the scale.


What you will find in the following pages can commute your sentence in that prison of fat. It can be your eleventh hour reprieve.

After working with obese patients for more than twelve years—and being a reformed fatty myself—I have a "magic" formula that is not magic at all.

The program described in this book is no panacea— BUT, it is the *easiest,* surest way to lose weight.

Rapidly.

*Safely.*

This is not a fad diet. You have a medical problem and it must be treated as such. The program must be carried out under a doctor's supervision. Go to him or her. You can't do it yourself. If for no other reason, because you need someone to guide you and reprogram you when you've reached your proper weight.

And you *will* reach your proper, desired weight.

My patients are somewhat disbelieving—incredulous is more the word—when I tell them that *getting their fat off is no problem.*

That's the easy part.

Following this regimen, *patients lose on an average of twenty to twenty-five—and sometimes more—pounds the first month.*

Yes, stay on this protein-sparing fast and your weight loss can be twenty, fifty, one hundred pounds, whatever you need to lose.

The weight comes off. It has to.

The hard part, the real goal, is to keep the weight off. The object of this program is not only to bring you down to a "normal" weight, but to keep you down there for the rest of your life.

A study done several years ago found that the backsliding rate for every diet it scrutinized was demoralizingly high. Of everyone who lost weight on any kind of diet, these researchers discovered that more than ninety-five percent put all the weight back on within twelve months.

This program has a far more encouraging story to tell. Of those patients I have seen again one year after they completed the protein-sparing fast and the behavior modification retraining, more than eighty percent have kept all or almost all of the weight off.

Let me repeat that.

*Eighty percent.*

Sorcery?

No. Self-motivation.

Self-motivation to get yourself together enough to try this program.

No data exists yet for claims of success that are medically meaningful, but I am fully confident that as the years pass, they will be published and they will confirm my own observations. You can become one of the happy statistics.

You have to want to lose weight enough to try my "Last Chance Diet." It will work for you. This is no hocus-pocus nor "who-knows-why-the-weight-comes-off-it-just-does" approach.

I will tell you how and why you will reduce.

You also need self-motivation to allow yourself to be reprogrammed into good nutritional eating habits that will keep you thin for the rest of your life. But good eating habits are a lot easier to pick up when you're a dress size 8 or a pants waist 32.

Not only is this your "Last Chance Diet," it can and should be your last diet. Period.

DR. ROBERT LINN

# 1

## *Why You Get Fat*

THIS COUNTRY has a food fixation. Take it back to those Pilgrims and Squanto the Indian, who gave thanks for the first harvest by having a food orgy.

Food. Food. Food. Our holidays are all associated with some gross overindulgence or another. The Thanksgiving turkey. The Christmas goose and plum pudding. The Easter eggs and chocolate rabbits. Fourth of July barbecues. Labor Day picnics. Somehow our national mentality is such that more food means we're going to have a better time.

Pick up a psychology book and it will explain how, as infants, food was one of our first associations with pleasure. When mother fed you, there was instant warmth and love. Food, then, became associated with those feelings of well-being.

Then food became a reward. "Be a good kid and I'll give you a cherry lollipop." You were commanded to clean your plate or have no dessert.

Sweets for the sweet. Send your loved one a box of chocolates.

You know how you got fat. For some it was a slow process. While you were hardly aware of it, your level of activity decreased, but you didn't compensate by cutting down on calories. When Lawrence, a patient of mine who dropped forty pounds on my program, was in high school, he lifted weights. But after his marriage, the most he lifted was slices of bread to his mouth. He admits he was a "breadaholic." Over the years, the weight went on.

Or the change in activity might have been far more subtle, as was the case of the secretary who switched from a manual typewriter to an electric. She found that she had gained five pounds in a year without changing her eating patterns.

Sometimes it's emotional stress. One of my patients started putting on weight after her best friend from childhood was seriously injured in an automobile accident. The friend's brain was damaged, changing her from a vibrant adult to a backward child. My patient told me: "I'm the kind who instead of worrying the weight off just started eating and ballooned out in no time at all."

Some psychiatrists will tell you that there are people who use their fatness as a barrier to having to cope with sex. Or that for others obesity is related to obsessive-compulsive behavior. An obsessive-compulsive person tries to control everything and everyone—including himself or herself. We all know that absolute control is an impossibility. So, say the psychiatrists, an obsessive-compulsive will mutate "control" into total *lack of control*. This type of person becomes fat because he or she has abandoned all attempts to curb gorging.

Boredom and sexual frustrations may have led to your overweight and fatigue is often a factor. Being tired often causes overeating. The higher centers of your cerebrum are also tired. You can't resist temptation when you're tired, it's harder to discipline yourself.

Despite what you might think, there is no additional physical need for more energy, more food, when you're fatigued. Your fat is an energy depot. You have the energy already stored.

Regardless of the reasons for your being fat what is important now is taking the weight off and keeping it off.

Contrary to popular notion, fat people aren't happy people, with the possible exception of Santa Claus. They will often attempt to hide their anger with a happy, outgoing demeanor, but that is only a mask.

When we snap the "before" pictures of my patients, they are often captured as unsmiling and glum, shoulders stooped as if they want to hide within themselves. These are different people in the "after" pictures, happy, with head held high.

The obese person often doesn't like his or her appearance and doesn't like himself or herself. They want people to accept them on a personality basis because the fat person is certain of not being accepted on a physical one. In fact, the jolly fat person is really a very angry individual underneath the adipose.

Glancing through the answers in the self-improvement booklet that my patients are asked to fill out when they begin the program gives you some indication of the hostility that is embedded in those layers of fat.

Asked to complete the sentence "My life is . . . ," some will write ". . . a flop" or ". . . a mess." "I'm annoyed by . . ." is answered by others with ". . . people who tell me to lose weight." One woman wrote she was annoyed by her husband.

But many of them "dream" of being thin, and complete "if only . . ." with ". . . I could lose thirty pounds in a day."

You know how you got fat, but you don't have to stay fat. What you have before you is the last chance diet. First decide, do you want to lose weight, undoubtedly increase the length of your life, make yourself less susceptible to certain diseases—heart disease and diabetes, to name only two—have more energy and feel better? Do you *really* want to lose weight?

You can.

## PERILS OF OBESITY

The problem of obesity is not just one of vanity. Sure, in our society where attractiveness and sensuality are often coupled with slimness, it is desirable for your own feeling of self-esteem to have your weight down. Sexy is slim to us. But there is much more to the perils of obesity than vanity.

Fat can mean early death.

Why do you think overweight people have to pay higher life insurance premiums? The answer is found in the actuary tables. They show a significant negative correlation between overweight and longevity. You may be cutting years off your life by putting pounds on your body.

There is different opinion on the subject, but many doctors now agree that fat people are more predisposed to disease. There is little disagreement, however, on the connection between obesity and diabetes, hypertension, and higher blood fat levels.

You greatly increase your chance of getting diabetes and getting it sooner by being fat. Your blood pressure more than likely will be higher as a fat person. Add the high fat levels to those factors and you are increasing your likelihood of getting a coronary artery disease.

As a fatty, the cards are stacked against you.

Nor does it end there. As C. F. Gastineau, M.D., put it, ". . . the relation between obesity and a given disease, if it exists, may not be linear; and because of practical difficulties in measuring degrees of obesity and excluding other risk factors, the hazards of being obese may not be readily proved.

"Some of these hazards are clear."

He goes on to point out the relationship between obesity and impairment of ventilation and congestive heart failure. Also, should you need surgery, your chances of surviving are lessened by the fat the doctor has to work through.

As you get older, that extra weight is going to take its toll in a quite mechanical way. Your joints were designed to take a certain amount of stress and weight. Being overweight means they have to deal with more than is optimum for them. After a while, degenerative joint diseases may develop.

These are the physical perils of obesity. Very real. Very frightening. But the vanity aspect should not be discounted either.

Obesity may very well cause a disease of the ego. Being fat very often destroys your self-esteem. You value yourself less because you're fat. That may seem, as you read it, to be ridiculous, but it does happen.

Slimming down may not cause a complete change in

your life—just as using that certain toothpaste isn't really going to change anyone's love life—but you may find it easier to cope with some things, because by losing weight you have proved to yourself you can set out with a goal and accomplish it.

Don't put off giving yourself the pep talk, giving yourself the motivation, pushing yourself to get started. This time, with my Last Chance Diet, you can make it. You can reach your goal.

Give yourself this gift—and get going.

# 2

# *Why You Stay Fat*

I<small>F</small> "<small>MALFUNCTION</small>" of your head—your mind and emotions—got you fat, it could very well be that "defects" in your body are keeping you that way.

"Don't eat too much," you've been nagged.

"Cut down on sweets."

"Don't gorge."

"Don't binge."

"The best exercise is pushing yourself away from the table." A cacophony of commands and counsel.

Women's magazines, always alert for an article that will fill space and sell copies, often come up with some sage advice along such lines.

All true, but not the whole truth. This advice is enough off the mark to keep you in a perpetual state of anxiety and depression.

"If all it takes is will power," you anguish, "then there

must be something wrong with me. I just don't have the will power to say no. I just can't stop eating."

When you do stop eating, or cut down, it seems hard for you to lose any appreciable amount of weight. Depression feeds on depression.

However, there may be something of which you're not aware. Something you may have suspected, but no one confirmed.

It is more difficult for you, a heavy person, to lose weight than it is for someone slimmer.

It has been found that your overweight body is a different piece of machinery than one of normal weight. Those far-too-many pounds overload your body and modify it, so it is physically more difficult for you to diet.

There are several contributing factors to this phenomenon, but one of the major villains is insulin, the hormone which allows sugar in the bloodstream to be used as energy.

The latest theories have insulin as the "transmitter" of glucose to the brain as well as other tissues. The insulin enables the sugar to get through the body's cell walls so that it can be "eaten" and used.

Obviously, insulin is necessary for you to function.

But, unhappily for the obese person, insulin has two nasty characteristics which make the dieting dilemma even more difficult.

First, insulin is "lipogenic." That means it's fat-producing. If there's something you don't want to encourage when trying to lose weight, it is a substance that promotes more fat.

The second characteristic of insulin which bodes no good for the dieter, is its "antilipolytic" quality—it works against fat's being broken down.

Talk about a two-edged sword—producing fat *and* retarding its breakdown. Having more insulin than absolutely necessary, it would stand to reason, is not desirable for the dieter. Insulin can only make weight reduction an even harder chore.

Now for the really bad news.

If you're fat, you (more than likely) have a resistance to insulin—you need more insulin than a slender person to get the same job done.

This resistance, it is believed by some scientists, is caused by the abnormal size of the fat cell in a heavy person. You may be fat for two reasons. One, you may have more fat cells than normal—something brought on while you were maturing; or, two, your fat cells are larger than usual. It's these large cells that cause the development of insulin resistance.

Studies have found that you might need as much as two to three times more insulin than someone of normal weight to take the same amount of sugar from the bloodstream—either to be stored or to be used as energy. If your body needs two to three times more insulin to function properly, that also means two to three times more of a substance that retards your ability to break down fat, while at the same time helping the manufacture of fat. This faster extraction of glucose from the bloodstream means that the heavier person gets hungrier sooner.

So from the start you are fighting a losing battle with yourself because your insulin level is higher than normal. A battle that has nothing to do with your head, your emotional reasons for eating, except they are probably what got you fat to begin with.

There are many vicious circles in the weight reduction process. These circles have the "fat getting fatter" or at least staying fat.

Take, for example, the internal stress cycle.

Everyone has stress, some minor, some major.

Stress may be having to drive through a wall of rain, surrounded by maniacs in other cars who think they are driving in the Grand Prix.

Stress might mean striving to make a deadline at the office. Keeping the kids from disemboweling each other. Rushing for a bus. Losing your car in a mammoth shopping center parking lot. Worrying about bills. Planning a big social event. Fretting over a business deal.

Stress is a part of life, an integral part of twentieth century life, in which speed and worry are of the essence.

Your body reacts to stress by pouring adrenalin into your bloodstream. This adrenalin is a kick, a trigger which gets the sugar stored in the liver out and ready to be used as energy. It's that energy that gives you the punch to respond to stressful situations.

When you're under stress, your blood sugar level goes up.

That wouldn't be detrimental for the dieter, except that the cycle has only just begun.

Your body reacts to the additional sugar: "Whoa, get that extra sugar out of the blood. There's too much floating around."

Off goes another trigger—from the brain to the pancreas. Guess what the pancreas produces?

Right. Insulin.

Out comes insulin to pull the excess sugar into storage. But you need more insulin—with its two-edged blade—to accomplish the maneuver. And there you are—stress to adrenalin to insulin to difficulty in losing weight.

One purpose of the protein-sparing fast is to lower the production of insulin—which it does, effectively and surely.

I will explain this in more detail in the chapter on how my program works, but, put simply, your energy source on the fast is not glucose. You will be using very little of this sugar. Instead, you will be relying on your own fat stores. With the reduction in glucose in the body, there is a corresponding reduction of insulin production. The pancreas is not as stimulated. You thereby virtually eliminate a barrier to rapid weight loss.

Recently there has been much publicity given to a condition known as hypoglycemia. Basically, hypoglycemia means that a person has lower blood sugar than is normal or desirable.

It has bizarre symptoms, ranging from anxiety and irritability to convulsive seizures.

The present controversy lies in just how prevalent this condition is. And here we get into a classical medical numbers game.

To have true "chemical" hypoglycemia, you have to run blood sugar levels of forty-five milligrams percent or lower. There are very few people who run this low, causing many medical "experts" to pooh-pooh hypoglycemia as a rare condition, not worth the publicity.

What these experts refuse to recognize is the frequency of "functional" or relative hypoglycemia.

You may have a blood sugar level that's considered normal, let's say 110. You feel fine at 110. But let's also say that you have sudden plunges where your level will go from 110 to sixty-five in an hour. Now, according to the medical texts, sixty-five is still in the normal range, but that plunge may give you the same symptoms that a true hypoglycemic has—fatigue, short temper, dizziness, etc. Where you felt good at 110, you feel lousy at the lower level, even though it's "normal."

There is a way to overcome the symptoms—to eat. You strain to bring your blood sugar back up to where you feel good. You have a craving to eat. So you do eat—candy, cake, anything to give you a sugar lift.

But, here's another one of those vicious circles. Putting

more sugar into your blood stimulates the pancreas and
—lo and behold—out comes that villain, insulin.

Besides more insulin, you're also getting more calories,
and eventually they start to make their presence known
—right around your waistline.

I have found that some sixty per cent of the people
who come to me have a relative hypoglycemia. Their
eating "urges" are eating "needs." Because of this condition, this fast is the perfect program for them. It is one
program where they aren't taking glucose dives that keep
them feeling miserable. I've often been told by patients
that they never stuck to other diets because they made
them feel so awful. Their rationale was they would
rather be fat than feel terrible. This problem on the
protein-sparing fast is rare.

The other side of the blood-sugar coin is diabetes.

This is the disease where there is too much sugar in
the blood because the insulin level is low or you have
become resistant to it. Your tissues are unable to use the
sugar without insulin to pass it through the cell membranes. Initially many diabetics show a low blood sugar
level.

Diabetes is a genetic or familial disease. In other
words, you may have an inherited tendency toward it.

A link between obesity and diabetes has been estab-
lished. Obesity often causes the premature development
of the disease. If you're fat and you have a diabetic inclination, the disease will develop much earlier in life.

Now look what happens. A potential diabetic may have the hypoglycemic syndrome—he has drops in blood sugar. He eats to feel better. He gets fat. And he brings his diabetes on sooner.

Patient after patient comes into my offices with a history of diabetes in his family. The patient is a relative hypoglycemic. I have to tell them that unless they get that excess poundage off, if they stay fat, they can look forward to diabetes within a very few years.

Diabetics who are taking insulin at the beginning of the program can often control their disease just by their diet after the extra weight is taken off. They no longer need to take insulin or the hypoglycemic agents that are now suspected of causing heart attacks.

Once these diabetics have gotten their weight down, their resistance to insulin disappears. So the small amount of insulin the diabetic does produce can be used more effectively. This does not happen in all cases— when it does it is limited to people who became fat as adults.

Sometimes you want to get that extra weight off for reasons of vanity. Our society is a lot less fun and exciting for a fat person. If you believe that "everybody loves a fatty," then you probably still believe the world is flat.

Thin is "in." You know that.

But you also know by now that you have to reduce because overweight is a disease. You must purge yourself of this illness to feel better—and to live longer.

Being fat doesn't affect just your outside. It changes your insides, too. One study found that people who became obese as adults can undergo twenty-seven different metabolic changes.

One more incentive for losing weight—as if you don't have enough already—is that once you get your weight to where it should be, these abnormalities disappear with your excess pounds. You should lose your resistance to insulin and your whole metabolic make-up may fall back into place.

Some of these metabolic changes are overlooked or discounted because they don't rate high or low enough in the medical numbers game.

The important thing to keep in mind is that although you have eaten yourself to a point where your body is working against your losing weight, the protein-sparing fast end-runs these roadblocks.

As you will find, your major energy, most of your fuel, while you are on the fast is not glucose, the sugar which causes your problem. You will lose weight rapidly. Twenty, fifty, one hundreds, two hundred pounds—the amount of weight you need to lose doesn't matter. You may be certain you can lose it all!

Once your body machinery is functioning properly and efficiently again, you will be able to modify your thinking on food. When you adopt new eating patterns—if you're like the overwhelming percentage of my patients—you will keep your weight off.

REPEAT: Being obese alters your body machinery. More likely than not, you have a resistance to insulin, a hormone that encourages fat production while discouraging the breakdown of fat. By having this resistance to insulin, you have to produce more of it.

You might also be a relative hypoglycemic, a condition that causes you to eat more to feel better physically. These are but a couple of the ways that being fat is keeping you fat.

After years of studying obesity, I believe that the protein-sparing fast is the most effective and safe program I know for eliminating these barriers, thus making weight reduction a far easier process.

# 3

## Dr. Linn's History

M<small>Y NURSES</small> are slim.

I'm slim.

What patient is going to believe that a doctor can help with a weight problem if the helper can't cope with his own problem? Slender nurses are a good reminder that you can be that way, too.

But, frankly, not all my nurses are svelte when they're hired. Very often, they too have weight problems. However, they are put on the program immediately and the weight comes rolling off. Talk about fringe benefits!

It is not a bad thing for a nurse—or for that matter a doctor—to know firsthand what it's like to be heavy. People who have never had to worry about their weight just can't understand the anguish of dieting and obesity.

I know.

41

I was fat.

It's not an atypical tale.

Like so many others, it started at mother's bountiful table. Mother was a master at homemade noodles—round ones, oblong ones, square ones, unbelievably delicious. And she never let me or my two brothers leave that table as long as there was something on it.

Added to that, I was, as a popular song puts it, a "junk food junkie." I could rhapsodize on the relative merits of French fries, pizza, crackers, cookies.

The few-too-many pounds began to make their unwelcome appearance when I was still in high school.

More were added during my days at the Philadelphia College of Osteopathic Medicine, from whence I graduated in 1959. The numbers on the scale became even more unfriendly while I interned in Michigan, and later when I returned to the Philadelphia area to set up general practice.

Then, one day it happened. Two hundred and thirty-five pounds had settled rotundly on my five-feet eleven inches. I was thirty-two years old, looked ten years older, and was fat.

My weight, an obvious problem, annoyed me, but not enough for me to do anything about it. Not until, that is, one frying day on the golf course when I was hitting eight or nine over par. I had just finished the seventeenth hole and was meandering over to the eighteenth tee when my heart started tom-tomming as if I'd just run a mile in under four minutes.

Dizzy and anxious, I abandoned the course in favor of the emergency room.

The cardiologist there calmed me down. "Right now" he said, "I don't think you have anything more than an anxiety reaction, but you'd better get some of that weight off."

Doctor, heal thyself!

That was ten years ago. And I, like so many other Americans, had the unenviable task of figuring out how to do it.

I turned to the medical texts, only to find the diet literature primitive and depressing.

I began to experiment on myself. One type of dieting versus another—until finally, six months later, I was down to 165.

I know what it means to be fat. And I know how hard it is to diet—and to keep the weight off. Or at least, how hard it used to be. Ten years ago, George Cahill had not begun his association with ketones and George Blackburn knew as much as I did about protein-sparing—nothing. But that was ten years ago. Do yourself a favor—come out of the Dark Ages of Dieting. Protein-sparing fasting is the weight-control program of today, the final quarter of the twentieth century.

# 4

## Diet Fads and Their Fallacies—1

CHANGE YOUR eating pattern—by eating only yoghurt, ice cream or lollipops—and you will lose weight. Temporarily.

Fad diets do work for that short, exhilarating, hey-look-Ma-I've-lost-five-pounds-in-a-week period. But if you've ever tried restricting your eating to bananas and milk, or yin and yanged yourself to anemia on the zen macrobiotic diet, you probably know that you do lose weight—but not much and not for long.

In no time at all these monotonous diets—including low carbohydrate-high protein ones—become boring. You soon tire of these food games. And you find it's taking too long to lose an appreciable amount of weight—the weight you need to lose. In short order, you're back to your old destructive eating habits, and one more fad diet has hit the garbage heap.

47

Unfortunately for fad dieters, not only do these programs not work, but they may even be dangerous. Let's take a few pages to discuss some of the perils and pratfalls of other programs.

## PILLS

It has been estimated that Americans spend some $16,000 a minute for diets and weight-loss gimmicks. It's not that fat people are any more gullible or more easily conned than thin ones, but their willingness to fork over cash for every hoked-up, snake-oil concoction or vague promise is an indication of the degree of desperation the obese person suffers.

There is a whole slew of diet pills, ranging from the much-abused amphetamines that need a doctor's prescription to the Miracle-Through-the-Mail variety.

These mail-order pills, which for the most part probably present no danger, also do not offer much hope of weight reduction. On the whole, the most effective thing about these pills are their advertisements.

Take the case of something called Anapex Diet Plan Tablets. Back in 1970 it was hardly possible to pick up a true confession or movie magazine without being exhorted that you could lose "Eighty-five pounds of ugly fat in two short months." At the same time readers were told they would be "permitted as many meals as you wanted, eating as much or more than you ever did." Furthermore, the ad promised that the Anapex plan had a "100 percent success" rate.

As unbelievable as Anapex sounded, as ridiculous as its claims appeared to be, almost nine million pills—forty-three thousand bottles at $5.98 each—were sold in three and a half months in New York State alone.

At least one person was skeptical of Anapex claims. The New York State Attorney General's office forced the pill off the state's market and levied the president of the company with a $2,000 fine.

In the course of the litigation, a detailed analysis of this alleged weight-reducing pill was offered.

It was found that Anapex contained a local anesthetic which is believed to suppress the appetite by coating the mucous membranes of the stomach. Another one of its "miracle" ingredients was a bulk producer which absorbs water and supposedly reduces hunger contractions. Both chemicals are often found in this type of pill. Whether either ingredient does what it is supposed to do is questionable. Indeed, in the case of the bulk producer, it has been pointed out that even if it did work, did reduce hunger contractions, overweight people eat although they are not hungry. Cutting down on the number of hunger contractions won't do much to appease the psychological part of appetite that must be differentiated from hunger, the physiological condition.

Another ingredient of many of these over-the-counter pills is B vitamins. They're included not because they are going to help you lose appetite or weight, but for a reason that is often studiously avoided in the advertisements.

Many of these pill plans include—you guessed it—a

diet. The only way you'll lose weight is if you cut down on your food intake. So, ad promises to the contrary, to accomplish anything with these pills, you have to diet. Since many of the diets are of the low-carbohydrate or high-protein variety, the manufacturers thoughtfully include the vitamins which are often lacking in those diet regimens.

But there are times when these modified placebos can cause serious damage. One pill was removed from sale after it was shown that a person allergic to its main ingredient—a chemical causing drowsiness—could suffer severe complications.

More effective, but with the potential of greater harm, are the prescription pills that too many doctors have been too indiscriminately pushing for too long.

By far the most widely prescribed and used are the "pep" pills—called "uppers" or "speed" in the non-dieting, hip drug scene—taken as appetite suppressors. Besides putting a damper on your appetite, these pills will give you a sense of vigor and stimulation—you can go zinging through the most normal of activities with a feeling that all is right and better than usual. Which is why drug freaks like to "get off on" speed.

The "upper" that is dispensed most often for dieting is amphetamine. Discovered at the University of California in 1932, it has been in wide use since. However, the serious side effects and habit-forming quality of amphetamine has elicited the following statement from the American Medical Association:

"Their undesirable effects, including a tendency to produce psychic and, occasionally, physical dependence when used indiscriminately and in large doses, make their use hazardous."

Used over a long period, amphetamines have been known to produce something called "paranoid psychosis"—a mental illness in which the sufferer is in a constant fear of being persecuted.

Whatever the pros and cons of taking amphetamines over a short period of time for weight reduction, it must be remembered that they are only a crutch. They are a temporary abater of your appetite which at the same time keeps you from becoming depressed over dieting. But they are temporary. Once you stop taking them— which should be as quickly as possible—you are often back at the starting line, still a compulsive eater who is still a slave to food.

In short, it is more than likely that you've taken the very real risks of popping speed for only a temporary weight loss. To some people, the pills become a substitute for food. They equate the two so that when the appetite-suppressing effects of the pills wear off, the user is famished and goes on a binge.

After extended use, the pills no longer suppress your appetite, but you are still euphoric. The result is that you eat, gain weight, but don't feel guilty about it. I have patients come to me after being on Dexedrine for years. They look like the Goodyear blimp and can't understand why the pills didn't take their weight off.

Taking pills will often make you forget what will power is. You don't need will power when on amphetamines, because you have no desire to eat. Go off the pills and you have to rebuild your control back to the level it was before you started.

Amphetamines come packaged under a variety of names with a variety of other ingredients included. Back in the Fifties, the most common type was Dexedrine. Today various amphetamines or amphetamine derivatives enjoy popularity under such names as Pondimin, Tenuate and Fastin.

Pondimin (also sold as Ponderax) had been selling over the counter in England and the West Indies before it arrived here. It promised that after three weeks your metabolism would change, so that carbohydrates would no longer be converted to fat. Here at last, it would seem, was the Holy Grail of dieting—eat junk and be thin anyway.

Unfortunately, as could be expected, Pondimin was not without its problem side effects: dry mouth, diarrhea and sudden, unexpected onslaughts of drowsiness at the most inopportune times. (With droll humor, the British pharmaceutical house described this side effect as "lack of suppression of paradoxical sleep"—letting the consumer have to puzzle out the meaning of that one!)

Diarrhea could be so severe that in one case, a surgeon

had to stop taking the pill because he found he was interrupting delicate operations to take flight to the bathroom.

Fastin has been known to reduce your sex drive, and Tenuate has caused some near sleepless nights because it puts you up so far, you can't get down.

Some of the side effects from just normal use of amphetamines, according to the AMA, can be "nervousness, restlessness, tremors, insomnia, an irregularly fast heartbeat, high blood pressure, overdilation of the eye, and gastronintestinal upsets."

Another class of pill often used in dieting are metabolic medicines, such as thyroid pills, which serve to speed up your metabolic rate. A higher metabolic rate means more fuel is needed to keep it going.

However, taking thyroid for dieting should generally be avoided, as it can induce serious changes in your entire metabolic system.

And then there are the diuretics, otherwise known as water pills. They will bring on a rapid weight loss when you first start taking them, but of course that weight is all water, not fat. Sometimes doctors will prescribe them to give the patient a psychological boost, to give them a fast loss as a motivator for staying on a diet.

On the protein-sparing fast, carbohydrates, which act as a dam for body fluids, are eliminated. With them goes the need for diuretics.

There are also natural diuretics, such as caffeine. Drinking coffee will have the same effect, to a degree, as taking a diuretic pill.

# 5

## *Diet Fads and Their Fallacies—2*

## INCHES-OFF CONTRAPTIONS

THE PROMISES sound wonderful. The before-and-after pictures look promising. It's not pounds, the ads rave, it's inches you need to lose. Strap on our super-duper, can't miss belt/weight/sweat suit/electrical monstrosity and watch the inches disappear.

You'll have just as much chance of success with these phony inch reducers as the Indians had against John Wayne. The only way you're going to get inches off is by toning them up with the exercise program that the manufacturers of these contraptions so thoughtfully include. One study, in fact, put two sets of prisoners through a controlled exercise program. One set wore sauna shorts—kind of a rubber sweat suit—that were being advertised under a variety of names, all promising

# ENERGY EQUIVALENTS

The number of minutes required at the activities listed to expend the caloric energy of food items shown below.

|  | Caloric Content | Lying Down | Walking | Riding A Bicycle | Swimming | Running |
|---|---|---|---|---|---|---|
| *Beverages, Alcoholic* | | | | | | |
| Beer, 8 oz. glass | 114 | 88 | 22 | 14 | 10 | 6 |
| Gin, 1½ oz. jigger | 105 | 81 | 20 | 13 | 9 | 5 |
| Martini, 3½ oz. cocktail | 140 | 108 | 27 | 17 | 13 | 7 |
| Old Fashioned, 4 oz. glass | 179 | 138 | 34 | 22 | 16 | 9 |
| Rye whiskey, 1½ oz. jigger | 119 | 92 | 23 | 15 | 11 | 6 |
| Scotch whiskey, 1½ oz. jigger | 105 | 81 | 20 | 13 | 9 | 5 |
| Wine, 3½ oz. glass | 80 | 65 | 16 | 10 | 8 | 4 |
| *Beverages, Nonalcoholic* | | | | | | |
| Carbonated Soda, 8 oz. glass | 106 | 82 | 20 | 13 | 9 | 5 |
| Ice cream soda, chocolate | 255 | 196 | 49 | 31 | 23 | 13 |
| Milk, 8 oz. glass | 166 | 128 | 32 | 20 | 15 | 9 |
| Milk, skim, 8 oz. glass | 81 | 62 | 16 | 10 | 7 | 4 |
| Milk shake, chocolate | 421 | 324 | 81 | 51 | 38 | 22 |

| | Caloric Content | Lying Down | Walking | Riding A Bicycle | Swimming | Running |
|---|---|---|---|---|---|---|
| *Desserts* | | | | | | |
| Cake, 2-layer, 1/12 | 356 | 274 | 68 | 43 | 32 | 18 |
| Cookie, chocolate chip | 51 | 39 | 10 | 6 | 5 | 3 |
| Ice cream, 1/6 qt. | 193 | 148 | 37 | 24 | 17 | 10 |
| Gelatin, with cream | 117 | 90 | 23 | 14 | 10 | 6 |
| Pie, apple, 1/6 | 377 | 290 | 73 | 46 | 34 | 19 |
| Strawberry shortcake | 400 | 308 | 77 | 49 | 36 | 21 |
| *Fruits, Fruit Juices* | | | | | | |
| Apple, large | 101 | 78 | 19 | 12 | 9 | 5 |
| Banana, small | 88 | 68 | 17 | 11 | 8 | 4 |
| Orange, medium | 68 | 52 | 13 | 8 | 6 | 4 |
| Orange juice, 8 oz. glass | 120 | 92 | 23 | 15 | 11 | 6 |
| Tomato juice, 8 oz. glass | 48 | 37 | 9 | 6 | 4 | 2 |
| *Meats* | | | | | | |
| Bacon, 2 strips | 96 | 74 | 18 | 12 | 9 | 5 |
| Ham, 2 slices | 167 | 128 | 32 | 20 | 15 | 9 |
| Pork chop, loin | 314 | 242 | 60 | 38 | 28 | 16 |
| Steak, T-bone | 235 | 181 | 45 | 29 | 21 | 12 |

## ENERGY EQUIVALENTS (Continued)

| | Caloric Content | Lying Down | Walking | Riding A Bicycle | Swimming | Running |
|---|---|---|---|---|---|---|
| *Miscellaneous* | | | | | | |
| Bread and butter, 1 slice | 78 | 60 | 15 | 10 | 7 | 4 |
| Cereal, dry, ½ cup, with milk, sugar | 200 | 154 | 38 | 24 | 18 | 10 |
| Spaghetti, 1 serving | 396 | 305 | 76 | 48 | 35 | 20 |
| Cottage cheese, 1 tbsp. | 27 | 21 | 5 | 3 | 2 | 1 |
| *Poultry, Eggs* | | | | | | |
| Chicken, fried, ½ breast | 232 | 178 | 45 | 28 | 21 | 12 |
| Chicken, "TV Dinner" | 542 | 217 | 104 | 66 | 48 | 28 |
| Turkey, 1 slice | 130 | 100 | 25 | 16 | 12 | 7 |
| Egg, boiled | 77 | 59 | 15 | 9 | 7 | 4 |
| *Sandwiches, Snacks* | | | | | | |
| Club | 590 | 454 | 113 | 72 | 53 | 30 |
| Hamburger | 350 | 269 | 67 | 43 | 31 | 18 |
| Roast beef, with gravy | 430 | 331 | 83 | 52 | 38 | 22 |
| Tuna fish salad | 278 | 214 | 53 | 34 | 25 | 14 |

| | Caloric Content | Lying Down | Walking | Riding A Bicycle | Swimming | Running |
|---|---|---|---|---|---|---|
| Pizza, with cheese, ⅛ | 180 | 138 | 35 | 22 | 16 | 9 |
| Potato chips, 1 serving | 108 | 83 | 21 | 13 | 10 | 6 |
| Cheddar cheese, 1 oz. | 111 | 85 | 21 | 14 | 10 | 6 |
| *Seafood* | | | | | | |
| Clams, 6 medium | 100 | 77 | 19 | 12 | 9 | 5 |
| Crabmeat, ½ cup | 68 | 52 | 13 | 8 | 6 | 4 |
| Halibut steak, ¼ lb. | 205 | 158 | 39 | 25 | 18 | 11 |
| Lobster, 1 medium | 50 | 38 | 10 | 6 | 4 | 3 |
| Shrimp, french fried, 1 serving | 180 | 138 | 35 | 22 | 16 | 9 |
| *Vegetables* | | | | | | |
| Beans, green, 1 cup | 27 | 21 | 5 | 3 | 2 | 1 |
| Carrot, raw | 42 | 32 | 8 | 5 | 4 | 2 |
| Lettuce, 3 large leaves | 30 | 23 | 6 | 4 | 3 | 2 |
| Peas, green, ½ cup | 56 | 43 | 11 | 7 | 5 | 3 |
| Potato, boiled, 1 medium | 100 | 77 | 19 | 12 | 9 | 5 |

to reduce your girth. The other set of prisoners did not wear the shorts. Results? Those who were lucky enough to wear the sweat-producing wonder garment lost no more than their cooler counterparts. No difference whatsoever.

If these devices don't help you, they certainly can work to your detriment.

Take one item that has been selling well for some twenty-five years—the Relaxicizor. If you were to believe the ads for this contrivance, you would be under the mistaken impression that the electricity that runs from the machine to your body will force your muscles to contract, thus firming up your body.

No such luck. What this distant relation to something you might see in a Boris Karloff movie may do, however, is cause heart failure, and according to one federal judge who heard testimony on it, contribute to "gastrointestinal, orthopedic, muscular, neurological, vascular, dermatological, kidney, gynecological and pelvic disorders." And just in case he missed something, the judge added to the list, the possibility that the Relaxicizor would exacerbate "epilepsy, hernia, multiple sclerosis, spinal fusion, tubo-ovarian abcess, ulcers and varicose veins."

The Relaxicizor was finally put on the prescription list by the Federal Drug Administration.

A device called Tone-O-Matic had a run-in with another federal agency, the Federal Trade Commission, this time on a false advertising complaint. "Whittle inches from your waist (firm up your thighs and hips, too)" the less-than-truthful ads read. The FTC took exception to the promise that a weighted belt was going to do all that. Moreover it found that the belt could do damage to some wearers.

Again, the only way to tone your muscles is through proper exercise. And exercise is a calorie consumer. The more you exercise, the more fuel you need to burn. By exercise, I don't necessarily mean sit-ups and push-ups There is enjoyable exercise, like swimming, tennis, bi cycle riding. Of course, one of the best forms of exercise is walking. I have considered having my patients strap on a pedometer to measure how much walking they do in a day. I encourage them to do more. Below is a chart showing some of the calorie equivalents of various types of exercise. It shows clearly how much exercise is needed to use up various types of food.

## CALORY EXPENDITURE FOR VARIOUS KINDS OF ACTIVITY *

TYPE OF ACTIVITY

CALORIES
PER HOUR †

*Sedentary*
Reading; writing; eating; watching television or movies; listening to the radio; sewing; playing cards; typing and miscellaneous office work and other activities done while sitting that require little or no arm movement.    88 to 100

*Light*
Preparing and cooking food; doing dishes; dusting; hand-washing small articles of clothing; ironing; walking slowly; personal care; miscellaneous office work and other activities done while standing that require some

CALORIES
PER HOUR †

arm movement; and rapid typing and other activities
done while sitting that are more strenuous.                    110 to 160

*Moderate*
Making beds; mopping and scrubbing; sweeping; light
polishing and waxing; laundering by machine; light
gardening and carpentry work; walking moderately fast;
other activities done while standing that require moderate arm movement; and activities done while sitting
that require more vigorous arm movement.                       170 to 240

*Vigorous*
Heavy scrubbing and waxiing; handwashing large articles of clothing; hanging out clothes; stripping beds;
other heavy work; walking fast; bowling; golfing; and
gardening.                                                     250 to 350

*Strenuous*
Swimming; playing tennis; running; bicycling; dancing;
skiing; and playing football.                              350 and more

* Adapted from Page L., and Finccher, L. J. *Food and Your Weight.*
  Home and Garden Bulletin No. 74, U.S. Department of Agriculture,
  1960, P. 4.
† Lower figures apply to women, higher figures to men. The figures
  include the metabolism at rest as well as for the activity.

# 6

## Diet Fads and Their Fallacies—3

B<small>ASICALLY DIETS</small>, excluding fasting, can be categorized in four ways—low calorie, low carbohydrate, high protein and high fat. All these Nirvana diets that hit the market with names like "No-Risk," "Prudent" or "Diet Revolution" are variations on one of these models.

There are two disadvantages to all of them. One is the amount of time needed to reach your weight-loss goal. Someone who needs to lose fifty, sixty, or even twenty pounds has to have the fortitude of a Daniel and the patience of a Job to stay on these diets to the very end. The temptation is constant and ever-present. There is always "tomorrow," when you'll eat less. And the reward of seeing your unwanted pounds evicted summarily is not present on these regimens.

The second disadvantage to these diets—and this can't be emphasized too strongly—is that nothing can take the place of medical supervision. No matter what you read. No matter what the advertising claims promise you.

You need a doctor to be carefully watching for silent disease, such as high blood pressure.

And just as crucial, you need a doctor for supportive therapy. He is someone who will encourage you to stay on a program and nudge you back to it when you stray.

Along these lines, those commercial weight-loss clinics that are beginning to open up around the country should be avoided. Although these establishments make a special point of advertising that clients will be "under medical supervision," this doesn't mean that you will be carefully watched by a doctor.

In fact, very often clients see a doctor but once or twice during the program. Why? Because these "clinics" aren't being run by a doctor. Instead, they may be owned by a shoemaker or a plumber who hires a doctor to come in once in a while. The "clinic" will also hire nurses and secretaries, but "medical supervision" at these places are a sham.

In May, 1976, The American Society of Bariatric Physicians warned that *"the casual administration by commercial clinics or other organizations where the supervision of patients by physicians is only cursory, can represent a serious threat to the health and welfare of the patient.* Severe unconventional approaches for the treatment of obesity should be reserved solely to specially trained and qualified physicians who personally monitor the progress of patients on a very frequent and regular basis. The administration . . . by anyone other than such a physician may threaten the very well-being of the patient."

Most of the variations of the four basic diet models have disadvantages beyond this that are peculiar to them. For instance . . .

## THE ONE-THOUSAND CALORIE DIET

Without doubt, the one-thousand calorie diet is the hardest, toughest, most painful kind of program to follow. You're hungry. And what stronger lure for falling off the wagon into the refrigerator than hunger?

Anyone can stay on a program for a week or two. But if you're following most of the low-calorie diet plans, a week or two means a loss of only a few pounds. Theoretically, a rule-of-thumb guide is that one pound can be lost in one week if you cut down on your daily calorie intake by 500. A two-pound loss in a week takes one thousand fewer calories a day. You would have to cut your daily calories by *four thousand* to lose eight pounds in a week.

This long, tortuous process leaves plenty of time for falling by wayside inns for a beer, a bowl of chili with a refried beans chaser, topped off with a triple banana split.

There is at least one motivating factor that can keep someone on a low calorie regimen, and that's sex. But other than someone who has sex as a strong motivator, anyone who stays on a one-thousand calorie diet until fifty or sixty pounds are lost merits attention in the *Guinness Book of Records.*

There are other objections to calorie-counting as a means of losing weight. For one thing, some scientists are now saying that there are different types of calories. A protein calorie is not the same as a carbohydrate calorie. Also, recent research has begun to question the belief that overeating is the sole cause of obesity. One study found that the fat people researched ate less than the thin people in the group, but remained fat. We've already discussed the changes that occur in your body when you gain weight which make it more difficult for you to lose weight. When you have those barriers to begin with, trying to persevere on a low calorie diet becomes a test of will no person should have to endure.

Low-calorie diets work in theory but not practice, because they are so difficult to stay on. One study, reviewing the success rate of a number of nutrition clinics, found that in general only thirty percent of the patients in these clinics lost twenty pounds or more. Only *nine* percent lost more than forty pounds!

## LOW CARBOHYDRATE DIETS

One of the earliest proponents of the low-carbo diet was an English doctor named John Yudkin. Dr. Yudkin's program, basically, was to limit your carbohydrates to fifty grams a day. He said that by doing this your calorie intake would also decrease by thirty-five percent.

There are two major disadvantages to this type of program.

First, it's a fairly tricky numbers game when you have to keep your carbohydrate count between fifty and sixty grams a day. Above sixty there may be a negligible weight loss or none at all, below fifty there can be considerable fatigue  So one misweighed piece of cheese or an overly generous slice of cantaloupe and you've loused up the dieting day.

But perhaps even more undesirable is the fact that a good portion of what you're losing to begin with is water. Then when you do start losing fat, your body replaces the lost water and you hit a plateau.

One variation of the low-carbo diet, the one to first become popular in the United States, was the Drinking Man's Diet. It was also called the Air Force Diet, the Airline Pilot's Diet and the Astronaut's Diet, much to the dismay of these groups. Basically it was a low-carbohydrate diet that let you drink alcohol. It's only been recently that the hidden danger in this regimen has been brought out. Scientists are beginning to find evidence that a high triglyceride—blood fat—level may be a more important factor in heart attacks than is a high cholesterol level.

And what is the biggest offender when it comes to raising your triglyceride level? Alcohol. If you have a tendency toward high triglycerides, alcohol will increase that likelihood. This is a silent phenomenon. You are not aware your triglycerides are going up—but your heart is aware of it.

It must also be remembered that when you drink and eat at the same time, the alcohol gets used first by the body for energy. The food you've eaten, will get "bumped" in favor of the alcohol—and will be put into fat storage.

A series of studies at the University of Ottawa has uncovered another problem with the low carbohydrate diet. Researchers there have found that such an alcoholic eating regimen may bring on hypoglycemia, by producing a below-normal blood sugar level. According to Harvard nutritionist Dr. Jean Mayer, "Many people who go on a weight-loss diet also increase their physical exercise, as indeed they should. Hard exercise increases our need for glucose and glycogen. Dieters who drastically reduce their carbohydrate intake and who continue to drink moderately and undertake a good exercise program may well be courting severe hypoglycemia."

## HIGH PROTEIN—HIGH FAT DIETS

Dr. Irwin Maxwell Stillman's Quick Weight Loss Diet, also known as the water diet, is perhaps the most famous of the high-protein diets.

Eat protein and drink lots of water. The problem here is monotony. Eating only protein very quickly results in superboredom. And superboredom very often forces even the most motivated person to abandon the diet.

The Stillman diet should be approached with utmost caution by anyone susceptible to high cholesterol levels.

This is mainly a diet of animal protein and fat—which translates into lots of cholesterol.

All these different diets—be they the one-food diet where you bore yourself into eating less by consuming only watermelon, or what have you, or be they of the Quick Weight Loss variety, represent part of the never-ending game that fat people play. Each new diet is a new head game. You pounce on it victoriously. Here at last is the magic combination for you, that will slim you down.

But they don't. And if they do take weight off you, it all comes back sooner or later.

This doesn't have to be. With this program, the pounds go so quickly that you don't have time to lose your precious motivation. And once you've bade those unwanted pounds farewell, that head that's given you so much trouble up to now, is sorted out, put into good working order and you are introduced to new feelings about food and new techniques of dealing with food. This is what other programs lack. They are temporary. This program is not, for it is multi-phasic. There is more to your weight-loss than those pounds disappearing— and that extra something is keeping the pounds off.

# 7

## Pep Talk

THE OVERWEIGHT problem is finally getting the wide attention and intensive research it deserves. One out of every five adults in the United States is overweight. Most of them will remain that way and die years earlier than their thin counterparts. Medical research constantly confirms the links between too many pounds and heart damage, diabetes, gall bladder ailments, and other metabolic disorders.

You know this.

Like most people, you've told yourself "It may happen to the other person but it won't happen to me."

Fear won't make you thin. People rationalize away their fears. Example? There is absolutely no doubt whatever that there is a direct relationship between cigarette smoking and your chance of dying of cancer, heart fail-

## AVERAGE WEIGHT OF AMERICANS [1]
### (in pounds according to height and age range)

#### MEN

| Height | | 15-16 | 17-19 | 20-24 | 25-29 | 30-39 | 40-49 | 50-59 | 60-69 |
|---|---|---|---|---|---|---|---|---|---|
| | | | | | Age range | | | | |
| Feet | Inches | | | | | | | | |
| 5 | 0 | 98 | 113 | 122 | 128 | 131 | 134 | 136 | 133 |
| 5 | 2 | 107 | 119 | 128 | 134 | 137 | 140 | 142 | 139 |
| 5 | 4 | 117 | 127 | 136 | 141 | 145 | 148 | 149 | 146 |
| 5 | 6 | 127 | 135 | 142 | 148 | 153 | 156 | 157 | 154 |
| 5 | 8 | 137 | 143 | 149 | 155 | 161 | 165 | 166 | 163 |
| 5 | 10 | 146 | 151 | 157 | 163 | 170 | 174 | 175 | 173 |
| 6 | 0 | 154 | 160 | 166 | 172 | 179 | 183 | 185 | 183 |
| 6 | 2 | 164 | 168 | 174 | 182 | 188 | 192 | 194 | 193 |
| 6 | 4 | . . . | 176 | 181 | 190 | 199 | 203 | 205 | 204 |

## WOMEN

| | | 97 | 99 | 102 | 107 | 115 | 122 | 125 | 127 |
|---|---|---|---|---|---|---|---|---|---|
| 4 | 10 | 97 | 99 | 102 | 107 | 115 | 122 | 125 | 127 |
| 5 | 0 | 103 | 105 | 108 | 113 | 120 | 127 | 130 | 131 |
| 5 | 2 | 111 | 113 | 115 | 119 | 126 | 133 | 136 | 137 |
| 5 | 4 | 117 | 120 | 121 | 125 | 132 | 140 | 144 | 145 |
| 5 | 6 | 125 | 127 | 129 | 133 | 139 | 147 | 152 | 153 |
| 5 | 8 | 132 | 134 | 136 | 140 | 146 | 155 | 160 | 161 |
| 5 | 10 | : | 142 | 144 | 148 | 154 | 164 | 169 | : |
| 6 | 0 | : | 152 | 154 | 158 | 164 | 174 | 180 | : |

[1] Adapted from table on average weights and heights, Build and Blood Pressure Study, Society of Actuaries, Chicago, 1959, vol. 1.[1]

ure, and a dozen other ailments. Yet look at how many millions of people continue puffing their way to earlier graves.

No, fear won't wash away those unwanted pounds.

If it would, you would have been thin again long ago.

What is going to work for you is the knowledge that apart from being a self-destructive physical habit, your extra pounds have made you look less attractive, feel less attractive, be less attractive. Your self image and your self esteem have suffered.

Away with all that.

Your pride in yourself can outweigh (no pun intended!) the momentary satisfaction of a candy bar. You'll become thin—you'll remain thin—and you'll love every minute of it.

Don't undervalue or underestimate the minutes. For every few pounds you drop could well add a few years to your life expectancy.

For many, the Last Chance Diet has been the first chance they have ever had to become attractively slim again.

For a few, my program was a lark. For the others, it was more difficult. It took determination, relearning and self-discipline. But for all who paid their dues by sticking to it, there was (and is for you) a definite weight loss. No lottery, this. Everyone, yes, *everyone* who pursues and perseveres this protein-sparing fast and the relearning program is a *sure* winner.

You don't get that kind of odds at the friendliest casino in Las Vegas.

# DESIRABLE WEIGHTS FOR MEN AND WOMEN
## AGED 25 AND OVER [1]
### (in pounds according to height and frame, in indoor clothing)

| Height [2] | | Small Frame | Medium Frame | Large Frame |
|---|---|---|---|---|
| **MEN** | | | | |
| Feet | Inches | | | |
| 5 | 2 | 112-120 | 118-129 | 126-141 |
| 5 | 3 | 115-123 | 121-133 | 129-144 |
| 5 | 4 | 118-126 | 124-136 | 132-148 |
| 5 | 5 | 121-129 | 127-139 | 135-152 |
| 5 | 6 | 124-133 | 130-143 | 138-156 |
| 5 | 7 | 128-137 | 134-147 | 142-161 |
| 5 | 8 | 132-141 | 138-152 | 147-166 |
| 5 | 9 | 136-145 | 142-156 | 151-170 |
| 5 | 10 | 140-150 | 146-160 | 155-174 |
| 5 | 11 | 144-154 | 150-165 | 159-179 |
| 6 | 0 | 148-158 | 154-170 | 164-184 |
| 6 | 1 | 152-162 | 158-175 | 168-189 |
| 6 | 2 | 156-167 | 162-180 | 173-194 |
| 6 | 3 | 160-171 | 167-185 | 178-199 |
| 6 | 4 | 164-175 | 172-190 | 182-204 |
| **WOMEN** | | | | |
| 4 | 10 | 98- 98 | 96-107 | 104-119 |
| 4 | 11 | 94-101 | 98-110 | 106-122 |
| 5 | 0 | 96-104 | 101-113 | 109-125 |
| 5 | 1 | 99-107 | 104-116 | 112-128 |
| 5 | 2 | 102-110 | 107-119 | 115-131 |
| 5 | 3 | 105-113 | 110-122 | 118-134 |
| 5 | 4 | 108-116 | 113-126 | 121-138 |
| 5 | 5 | 111-119 | 116-130 | 125-142 |
| 5 | 6 | 114-123 | 120-135 | 129-146 |
| 5 | 7 | 118-127 | 124-139 | 133-150 |
| 5 | 8 | 122-131 | 128-143 | 137-154 |

| 5 | 9  | 126-135 | 132-147 | 141-158 |
| 5 | 10 | 130-140 | 136-151 | 145-163 |
| 5 | 11 | 134-144 | 140-155 | 149-168 |
| 6 | 0  | 138-148 | 144-159 | 153-173 |

[1] Adapted from Metropolitan Life Insurance Co., New York. New weight standards for men and women. *Statistical Bulletin* 40:3, Nov.-Dec., 1959.[2]

# 8

## *Dr. Linn's Protein-Sparing Fast*

You've no doubt read it before, but to understand the protein-sparing fast, a short review of the basics of obesity is needed.

Fat is energy. Stored energy.

Your body requires only so much energy to function each day. The amount needed depends on how active you are. If you take in more energy—man's energy fuel is food—than your body can use, the excess will be very economically stored as fat.

If you push a pencil instead of a plow, spend most of the day behind a desk and the night in front of the television set, if your one major activity is guiding a shopping cart through aisles of fattening goodies, you are a sedentary person. Now if your optimum weight is one hundred pounds, with that limited activity, your body will burn up anywhere from one thousand to fifteen hundred calories a day. Take in more than that, and it goes right to fat, whether it entered your mouth as fat, carbohydrate or protein—the three basic foods. (You do store some carbohydrate, but only a small amount. There is also a limited protein storage.)

Losing weight, then, should be simple logic and simple mathematics. Cut down the amount of food you swallow and your body will be forced to use its fat reserve for energy.

Simple to understand, but not so simple to practice. Restricting your caloric intake is a slow and psychologically debilitating method of losing weight. A one-thousand-calorie diet cruelly allows enough to tempt you, but not enough to satiate you. It has been shown that the low-cal diet is the most difficult one to stick to. It takes so long to lose an appreciable amount of weight that only the strongest-willed can endure it.

Then, too, there are the previously discussed factors of insulin that make it more difficult for the obese person to lose weight.

All of which makes the concept of fasting—called by some the "ultimate diet"—so popular.

If cutting down on food causes you to lose weight, it would seem logical that eliminating food entirely should produce an even faster loss. Your only energy would have to come from within the body.

Which is what happens.

Unfortunately, however, on a total fast—where nothing but fluids are ingested—the energy source is not restricted to just your unwanted fat. Not only does your body dip into your fat stores for fuel, but also into your lean body mass—that's muscles, liver, kidneys, heart. On the total fast, which regrettably is becoming a national fad, only fifty per cent of the weight loss is fat and the rest is water and lean body tissue.

That's not the weight you want to lose. Fat is what you want to get rid of. Losing muscle and other lean body tissue is neither healthy, desirable, nor is it going to achieve what you want in the long run—permanent weight reduction.

Breaking down protein tissue is cannibalistic. You're "eating" your own "meat." You're not reducing the amount of fat pudgied over your body. Furthermore, this devouring of the protein mass puts the total faster into an undesirable condition known as "negative nitrogen balance."

Protein is the body's main source of nitrogen. When protein is broken down, nitrogen is excreted. By measuring the excretion, we can tell how much protein is being destroyed. When more nitrogen is being eliminated than taken in, you have this negative balance.

A total faster will tire easily. He's weak, has no stamina. He's virtually chipping away at his own muscles, which are the users of energy. Less muscle tissue means a diminished energy-using potential. Less energy used means more fat storage—a vicious obesity circle. Besides this, the total faster is apt to suffer from plummeting blood pressure when he gets up from a prone position. Vitamin and mineral deficiencies might result. The potassium levels in his body can be thrown completely out of kilter, leading to serious heart problems.

But just as "debilitating" to the total faster as these physical manifestations is what happens to him after he resumes eating. When the total fast is ended, the body immediately moves to return itself to nitrogen balance. It has an urgency to replace the lost protein tissue—and weight. *No matter what the total faster does, no matter how stingy he is with calories,* the scale goes careening upwards.

It has been found that for one pound of protein replaced, your weight could theoretically increase by as much as four pounds.

Figure it out.

If you lose twenty pounds the first month of a total fast, ten pounds will be lean body mass. Once you start eating, your weight could shoot up thirty pounds! A ten- or fifteen-pound gain in two or three weeks, however, is actually more likely.

It is only after a full month of total fasting that the percentage of protein loss begins to diminish significantly.

This depressing weight gain, although three-fourths of it is water, is not going to put the total faster into the frame of mind necessary to keep his weight down for the rest of his life, which should be the goal of any reducing program.

If you deprive yourself of food for an extended period of time only to have the pounds reappear practically overnight, it's little wonder that many fasters throw in their calorie counters and tear up their maintenance diets.

What is the "protein-sparing" fast, then? And more importantly, why does it work?

As on a total fast, no solid food is eaten. There is a major difference, however—a difference that takes weight off and keeps it off during the follow-up period when you are reprogrammed from bad eating habits to good ones. Habits that will keep you slim.

To inhibit the body from making protein a major fuel source and thereby creating a negative nitrogen balance, my patients are prescribed a predigested liquid protein formula that supplies them with all the necessary amino acids, the components of protein. As long as protein is being provided, only very minimal lean body mass is destroyed for energy.

This liquid, which I call Prolinn, is a formula composed of all the amino acids needed to form a protein molecule. They are present in the usable proportions necessary for this manufacture. With no carbohydrates or fats and fifteen grams of protein, a two-tablespoon portion of Prolinn contains sixty calories.

Under all conditions, protein is broken down in the small intestines into amino acids. These acids are then absorbed by the small intestines and transported to the tissues that need protein to function. Some of the

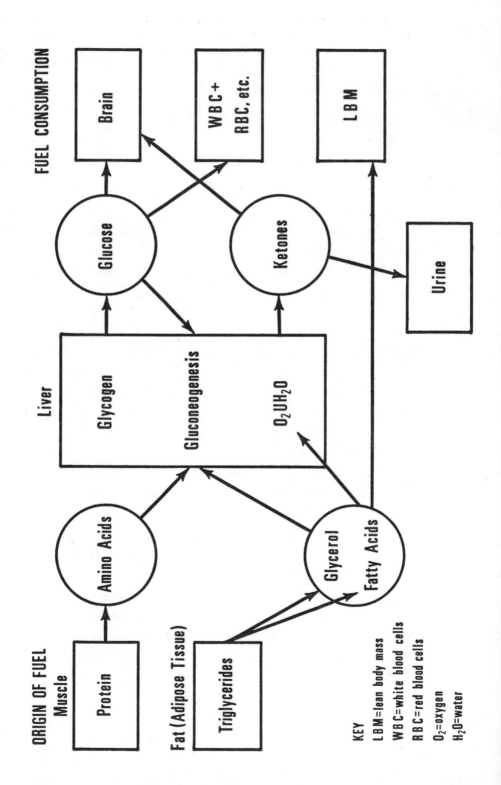

ORIGIN OF FUEL

FUEL CONSUMPTION

Muscle

Protein

Fat (Adipose Tissue)

Triglycerides

Amino Acids

Glycerol
Fatty Acids

Liver

Glycogen

Gluconeogenesis

$O_2 U H_2 O$

Glucose

Ketones

Brain

W B C +
R B C, etc.

L B M

Urine

KEY

L B M=lean body mass

W B C=white blood cells

R B C=red blood cells

$O_2$=oxygen

$H_2O$=water

excess amino acids are changed by the liver to glucose. A small amount of this glucose can be stored in the body as "glycogen." Any glucose above the glycogen storage capacity becomes fat. Glucose is the sugar the body uses for fuel under normal, nonfasting conditions.

Prolinn fills the protein requirements. Therefore, only five percent or less of the weight loss on this type of fast is protein, the other ninety-five percent being exactly what you want to see the last of—fat.

This also means that at the end of the fast, the body is in a relative nitrogen balance. Since the lean body tissue has not been used, there is no need for replacement.

Protein-sparing has the advantages of the total fast— the rapid weight loss—and none of the frightening disadvantages.

From the first day on the protein-sparing fast there is a weight loss. The patient doesn't need any carbohydrates or fats because he has an overabundant supply of fat energy. Someone of normal body weight has 135,000 calories of stored fat. He also has 24,000 calories of protein, 280 calories of glycogen in the liver, and 480 calories of glycogen stored in muscle. Compare that to the obese person, who has in store 360,000 fat calories, 28,000 protein calories, 280 liver glycogen, and 560 muscle glycogen. As you will note, the real calorie difference between a slim person and a fat one is in the fat storage. The other calorie storage is relatively close.

A gram of fat produces nine calories—nine units of energy—whether it comes from body fat or food fat. Your body doesn't care where the calorie comes from as long as it gets it. Once you are on the fast, an imaginary switch is thrown and the body turns to its own reserves.

Scientifically this is what happens on the protein-sparing fast:

After approximately twenty-four to forty-eight fasting hours, what little glycogen that has been stored in the liver is depleted. Deprived of food, your body must resort to something else for energy. By the time you've fasted for seventy-two hours, your body is no longer dependent on carbohydrates as its primary fuel source. It has gone to a nearly 80 percent dependency on stored fats, otherwise known as triglycerides.

When triglycerides are broken down, two products result. One is free fatty acids, the other, glycerol. Some of the free fatty acids go directly to the lean body mass for fuel. The remainder is partially oxidized by the liver into "ketone bodies."

It was not until 1967 that Oliver Owen, M.D., George Cahill, Jr., M.D., and others of Boston's Joslin Diabetes Foundation described how the body makes use of ketones. It was found that the brain can use these bodies as energy just as it does glucose. Until this study, it was believed that "ketosis"—this period of ketone production —was an unnatural and harmful state. It was also thought that glucose was the brain's only energy source.

On the contrary, it would seem that evolution provided man with a mechanism for switching body fuels in times when conventional foods are not available. Remember, man as a prehistoric hunter more than likely went through extended periods when game and food were scarce. He would have starved to extinction if his body had to rely on its meager carbohydrate stores.

As long as your body can use ketones and free fatty acids as "food," significant amounts of protein won't be destroyed for glucose production. When glucose is no longer the body's main fuel, the level of insulin—which I have already explained is a curse to the obese dieter—will drop.

Your body will use the ketones and free fatty acids for fuel rather than protein because they are a more economical energy supply. Your body is quite consistent in its desire for economy. You plunge into your fat to produce the ketones and fatty acids with such speed that some patients say they can practically see the fat "melting off." An exaggeration, perhaps, but just the kind of reward you need to keep you going. Fast, positive, and safe reinforcement. Six months or a year is a long time to keep motivation high, and plenty of time for discouragement unless you're losing rapidly. Once you have had the initial weight loss and you have settled down to a determined goal, your body will drop up to one-half pound of fat a day.

Studies have shown that on the protein-sparing fast, eighty percent of the fuel you need to function—and function as well and better than you ever have before—will come from the fatty acids and ketones. The other twenty percent comes from glucose that is manufactured by protein breakdown. But this is usual protein breakdown that you would have whether you were on the fast or not. Even when you're eating, you lose that much muscle tissue in a day, but it is immediately replaced by protein. When you're on this fast, it is replaced by the protein from the formula.

Ketone bodies produce a side effect that, happily, is very beneficial for the faster. Ketones can act as a natural appetite suppressant. No pills are needed to keep the hunger pangs curbed. Between eighty and eighty-five percent of my patients will have *no hunger at all*. Once you are able to eliminate the physical aspect of hunger, the psychological hangups of appetite are much easier to cope with. Hunger, it should be remembered, is the real, physical aspect of appetite. Another very important part of appetite is mental. Much of what you feel when you desire food is a state of mind.

The protein-sparing fast is without any major side effects. A very few people do experience minor ones, but they are strictly minor. Those that might occur will be discussed in detail in another chapter.

Why use Prolinn instead of lean meat or egg whites— once thought to be the most complete and best protein source?

By taking the formula, you are getting amino acids in the proportions needed for protein formulation. Prolinn is the most convenient and economical way to get the highest protein level possible.

Generally, women take four to five ounces of Prolinn

daily. Men get, on an average, seven to eight ounces. The daily Prolinn allowance depends on what weight the patient should be at the end of the fast. This program takes you down to where you should be. Too often diets and regimens will only get you to the neighborhood of your optimal weight and leave you with pounds still to lose. More often than not, you fail to finish the task. You get discouraged. And your weight goes spiraling upwards.

Sometimes the program must be modified slightly for hypoglycemics. They may have to increase their amounts of Prolinn by one or two ounces. I may also give them protein tablets. Occasionally I will even have them drink some skim milk—four ounces, twice daily.

Besides the Prolinn, you must take vitamin and mineral supplements to prevent deficiencies. One of the side effects of total fasting can be scurvy, the plague of sailors of an earlier era. The British earned the nickname "Limey" because English sailors stocked limes on long sea voyages to prevent this disease of the gums.

Patients are also required to take two to four grams a day of potassium and higher levels of folic acid than are found in nonprescription multiple vitamin pills.

On top of that, a minimum of one and a half to two quarts of fluids—water, coffee, tea or sugarless soda—must be drunk daily.

For awhile I was also prescribing baking soda to counteract any possible sodium deficiencies. But I noticed in my monthly tests that sodium levels in my patients were running from high-normal to high. I ran a formal study on fifty patients to determine whether a deficiency would occur without the sodium supplement. The results showed that patients *not* taking baking soda held normal levels. So I discontinued giving baking soda, much to the delight of my patients, who often complained of the taste.

When on the fast your uric acid level should be tested. If it is high, you must take medication to lower it.

Both uric acid and ketones are excreted through the urinary tract. When ketones are produced, the uric acid finds itself competing to be excreted. A uric acid backup results.

If the level is allowed to go too high, at the end of the fast, when ketones disappear, there is a rush of uric acid through the excretory system. A concentration in the kidneys may occur, causing the formation of kidney stones.

However, it is not difficult to control the uric acid level during the fast.

# 9

## *Dr. Linn's Protein-Sparing Fast (continued)*

Ｏ NE OF THE great advantages to the "Last Chance Diet" is its simplicity. As one patient remarked, "It's easier to do without than to do with little."

And it is.

There are no decisions to make. The decision not to eat—period—has already been made. There is no "Well, a little of this won't hurt. I'll just eat less tomorrow." You are not eating anything.

To simplify it even further, so you have minimal preparation and thought, I usually suggest that my patients mete out their Prolinn into a smaller container that holds the daily five, seven or eight ounces. They can then carry their day's supply wherever they go, along with a two-ounce cup for drinking. Prolinn does not require refrigeration.

You can go on with your daily activities without having to bother measuring. I have salesmen whose jobs include frequent business lunches. This program in no way interferes with their activities. They will usually take their Prolinn before or after the lunch and sit during their companions' meal and drink coffee, tea or no-cal soda.

My patients entertain, go to dinner parties, change their social and business lives only in the smallest ways, if at all. All the while, they are exuberant and filled with energy.

One young mother of a lively three-year-old complained after several weeks on the fast that she was often tired at the end of the day. She had started the program forty-eight pounds more than her weight at the time of her marriage.

"The fatigue," she told me, "is caused, in a way, by the fast, in that I have so much energy I go bounding out of bed in the morning. I do everything I can—cleaning chores I've put off for years. I guess the problem is, I *overdo*. But I can't help it, I'm so full of pep, I overtax myself."

After six weeks on the fast, the woman is, at this writing, within seven pounds of her wedding-dress size.

Albert Brown, a former colonel in the United States Army and onetime senior Army adviser to the State of Pennsylvania, came to me with some fifty extra pounds on his six-foot-five-inch frame. He had tried many different types of diets—even ordering the "miracle through the mail" pills. His most successful attempt at losing weight occurred when he endured the most grueling of spartan regimens while on duty in Vietnam.

For six months he denied himself all but a little food.

"One could do it there," he explained. "It was an area where there were no temptations. No family eating. Life was not going on at the mad dash you're usually accustomed to."

The base was also smothered in muggy, tropical heat.

"I had a strict physical regimen of running in the middle of the day when the temperature was ninety-eight or a hundred."

Colonel Brown managed to take off between thirty and forty pounds. But on his return to this country, the extra weight returned also.

Colonel Brown finished his protein-sparing fast more than a year ago. The fifty-two pounds he lost with my program stayed off.

"I'm trying to encourage the Army to start this program," he enthused not long ago. "The armed forces," he said, "have become alarmed by their overweight personnel to the point of issuing 'fat directives.'"

"The Army does have diet tables in some camps, but you're on your own. In the field such tables are not available. But with your program, someone can carry the formula out to the field easily. And there is no impairment to your thinking or a reduction of your activities."

(In an article in the magazine *Army* in April, 1976, Colonel Brown described his success with the Last Chance Diet. Ironically, he learned about the diet from a podiatrist, Dr. Elliott Bernstein, when he observed that

Bernstein, a fellow officer, had lost 50 pounds in two months, dropping from 238 pounds to 188, the desired goal for his age and height.

(Colonel Brown adds: "The soundest argument as to the superiority of Dr. Linn's method over others is that in only two months, without any great exertion, I lost more weight that I did with six months of a grueling monastic regimen in Vietnam.")

In recent months a furor has arisen over the need for fiber in the diet.

Fiber promoters claim that the decreased use of fiber in the American diet accounts for the high rate of heart disease and colon-rectal cancer in the United States. They base their claim on work done by a British scientist, Sir Denis Burkitt, who studied the Bantu tribe of South Africa.

Burkitt found that cancer of the colon and rectum and heart disease are almost nonexistent among the Bantus. It has been proposed that the Africans' diet, filled with fiber such as potatoes, yams, cabbage, nuts and roots, accounted for the low rate.

The theory goes that fiber, being insoluble, decreases the amount of time it takes all food to get through the digestive tract. The faster travel rate is supposed to get the irritants and fats linked to cancer and heart disease out of the intestinal tract before harm can be done.

Then, is going without fiber for an extended period of time—such as when on the fast—dangerous?

First, it should be said that the benefits of increasing your fiber consumption—whether it is really a "save your life diet"—is in serious question. In February, 1976, a panel of doctors and scientists from the American Association for the Advancement of Science, disputed many of the claims, saying that too much fiber can create nutritional deficiencies, possibly malnutrition, and flatulence.

Indeed, one doctor, Albert Mendeloff, a professor of medicine at Johns Hopkins University, pointed out that in the past thirty years, the incidence of colon-rectal cancer has actually remained the same. He further stated there is no evidence that the amount of fiber in the American diet has changed.

It would seem that the importance of fiber is being overplayed. The lack of it is just not a serious worry for the protein-sparing faster. I have had patients on the fast for up to nine months, losing as much as 160 pounds. Once they have resumed eating solid food, they have no problems with the digestive system.

Let's say there is truth to the idea that fiber is beneficial because of its faster travel rate, but it is not a factor in the protein-sparing fast. Since you're not eating any food, none of the irritants mentioned in the fiber diet will be in your digestive tract. Therefore, there is no need for something to move them through faster.

In fact, when a surgeon performs an intestinal bypass

—part of the intestine is "tied off" so that the absorbing surfaces are reduced by some ninety percent—and later undoes it, the patient returns very quickly to normal body functions. The gastrointestinal tract does not atrophy.

With protein-sparing, the trick is not getting the weight off. It must disappear. It does disappear. Rapidly.

I have a multi-phased approach to weight control— there is the key word. *Control.* This program is not only for weight reduction. That is easily accomplished, more easily than with any other regimen in existence.

The true purpose of removing your fat stores as quickly as possible is to prepare you for developing new eating habits. While I'll go into this in more detail in a later chapter, let me say here that it is far easier to re-program your attitudes toward eating and food when you're at a reasonable, proper weight.

I remind you again that the fasting program will take off all your excess weight. That is not the ultimate goal. Your goal is to keep the weight off. And that is the goal my patients—and you—can reach with the Last Chance Diet.

I have some patients who are literally afraid to begin eating at the end of the fast for fear of regaining their fat. Your re-entry into the world of eating is a slow, carefully planned program. Your fasting time serves an important function besides taking you down to a normal body weight. It dims your memory of food. You can then be re-educated to the point where a crispy green salad will be as tantalizing to you as a hot fudge sundae once was.

When she first came to me Susan S. was a twenty-one-year-old college student who had been fat all her life. When she came to me, she had one hundred and eighty pounds dumped on her five-foot-five-and-a-half body. Only once before had she been at all "successful" with a diet—a low calorie-high protein regimen that lasted from May until September. She lost thirty pounds—but kept them off only as long as it took her to find "the best chocolate I ever tasted" when she moved to London for a year. Zap. Susan was as fat as ever.

Now down two dress sizes after losing forty-four pounds (with just ten more to get off), Susan said, "You know, I don't feel like rushing out for an ice cream cone anymore. I'm dying for a piece of fruit. That will really be a treat. I've really changed my attitude about eating."

The behavorial modification aspect of this program is as important as the actual weight reduction. What good is losing your excess weight, only to put it right back on again? That my patients are successful in learning new eating habits is evidenced by the high percentage I have observed who do not regain their weight—*some eighty percent*. Compare that to the four percent success rate found with other diets. If you are serious about losing weight, you must also be serious about keeping it off.

REPEAT: The protein-sparing fast is a safe, nutritional regimen. It has the advantage of the total fast—rapid weight loss—without the disadvantages—destruction of lean body mass and rapid weight gain at the end of the fast

The protein-sparing fast is not easy, but it is far more certain than any other weight reduction and control program.

You need make no decisions about eating and food. The decision has already been made.

The program cannot fail. Only you can fail.

The rapid weight loss—an average of twenty to twenty-five pounds the first month and between sixteen and eighteen thereafter—is strong motivation for the patient to see the program through.

# 10

## *The First Days*

COLD TURKEY. It may seem brutal—having to walk into your doctor's office an eater, albeit an overeater, and walk out knowing that you will put no food into your mouth for one, two, three, possibly more months.

Sorry, but it's the only way.

The chain-smoker is only kidding himself when he says he'll quit by cutting down by a couple of cigarettes a day. A heroin addict isn't going to kick his habit by reducing the quantity of his daily fix.

It's all or nothing, so accept it. Get on with it and that surplus weight will evaporate. If the thought of not eating for so long—virtually depriving yourself of one of your favorite pastimes—is depressing, cheer yourself with the knowledge that *you will lose anywhere from seven to fifteen pounds in that first week.*

*With minimal fatigue, if any at all.*

My patients generally know what to expect when they come to my clinic. A friend on the program will have told them about it. They might have read about it somewhere. Or as in the case of the twins, Ruby and Roxie, they heard me outlining the program on a local radio show. It comes as no great surprise when I tell them that all their food will be taken away. There are, however, exceptions to everything. The L.'s were surprised.

Robert and Marsha L., after getting heavier and heavier together during their six and a half years of marriage, decided that the time had come to get thin together. Robert, at five-feet-eight, was overloading the scales at 189½ pounds. Five-foot-four Marsha was a hefty 161¾. Neither of them had ever really dieted, although Robert once had tried eating nothing but yoghurt for two weeks. He lost ten pounds, but put it all back immediately.

Definitely, the L.'s decided, the time had come to seriously lose weight. So Marsha checked the phone book for doctors specializing in the treatment of obesity and found my name.

"We didn't really understand Dr. Linn at first," Robert recounted almost sheepishly, twenty-eight and a half pounds later.

"He said, 'I'm going to take all your food away.' I thought he must be speaking figuratively."

The shock that I was speaking quite literally was not a deterrent and the L.'s went ahead with the program. Six weeks later, Marsha was down to 137, intending to keep going until she hit 123. Robert had just five more pounds to discard.

"I'm not worried about ever regaining the weight," Marsha said "I've seen both sides of the fence and I never want to be in the condition I was in before."

The L.'s, like everyone else, began Day One of the fast with the Prolinn. There is no "I'll start tomorrow." You've been doing that for too long as it is.

On your first visit, you get your first series of questionnaires and tests.

The first is a medical history, quite similar to the Cornell Indices—one hundred and thirty questions designed to facilitate giving the doctor an accurate picture of your health background while at the same time being comprehensible to him.

Questions like:

"Has your eyesight often blacked out completely?"

"Is your nose constantly stuffed up?"

"Does your heart often race like mad?"

"Do cuts in your skin usually stay open a long time?"

"Do you sweat a great deal in cold weather?"

"Do you have to get up every night and urinate?"

"Do you often get spells of complete exhaustion and/ or fatigue?"

"Did you ever have scarlet fever?"

"Has your doctor ever said you have a hernia?"

And so on.

After the questionnaire, you are given a complete physical—blood pressure, heart, lungs, abdomen, reflexes, etc.

For the next two weeks, be prepared to make frequent visits to your doctor's office. Besides giving you support and a chance to get any questions you might have answered, other tests must be run first—a five-hour glucose tolerance test (how you metabolize carbohydrates and sugar), an electrocardiogram, twelve different blood tests, including tests for uric acid, cholesterol, triglycerides, and others.

This is a medical program. It's imperative that the doctor knows what you are medically.

You're on your way to being a healthier human specimen than you've been in years.

Some patients initially have an atavistic fear of starvation. Something in them tries to insist that they will starve to death. That's nonsense, of course, since the body is being fed from within itself.

It doesn't take many days, however, for these patients to overcome this misinformed inner voice. Quickly they *emotionally* accept that the protein-sparing fast rather than being harmful is both safe and beneficial. Keeping that weight on is what is dangerous.

During my first talk with a patient on Day One I can often spot the person who isn't going to make it through the program—the one who will drop out, usually in the first few days. There are surprisingly few who do not make it—twelve percent at the most.

They are easy to spot. These patients already have excuses why the program must be modified for them, why they can't commit themselves to it completely.

"Can't I eat just on the weekend?"

"How can I not eat during business lunches?"

"I've got to taste what I cook for my family. The dishes won't come out properly."

Nonsense.

You don't have to eat to be social. Often your not eating seems a problem to non-fasters around you. They can't cope with your not joining them. But that's *their* problem. One of my patients, in an attempt to ease the discomfort of dining companions, will go to the salad bar in a restaurant and take a salad, which she won't eat. The mere appearance of her taking part in the meal seems to be enough to pacify the eaters.

Not eating at business lunches will give you more time to get your points across. Have some coffee, tea or diet soda.

And what difference does it really make if a dish is a little salty or needs a touch more oregano? Rita G., a five-foot-one housewife and bookkeeper, cooks three meals a day for her husband and five children. She has been on the protein-sparing fast for several months and has not had problems cooking rich pastas and extravagant desserts.

For awhile she stopped preparing fattening foods because she didn't think she could cook without tasting.

"I never make a dish exactly the same. With lasagne, that's a blending of cheese and spices. But tasting was my problem. I didn't just stop at one taste. Now there's nothing I can't make. Even the things that I like, I can now make and serve and not eat."

Mrs. G.'s weight is what is important to her. She was 204 pounds at the start of the program and has lost almost seventy pounds at this writing.

Your weight is what should be important to you. Your self-esteem. Your well-being.

Those first few days are the potentially dangerous ones. They are the time of adjustment. But the dramatic weight loss keeps people on this program. You have to lose and you should maintain close contact with your physician.

Again, *you will lose from seven to fifteen pounds in that first week.*

By the end of Week Two, you may have dropped a total of sixteen to eighteen pounds—which is where you can encounter your first major problem.

You must continually remind yourself not to set your own goals. You can depend on an average monthly weight loss—but not a weekly or daily one.

Plateaus are the dieter's bane. We will go into these demoralizers more fully in a later chapter, but often those first two astonishing weeks set you up for a let-down when and if you only lose three or four pounds in Week Three. The twenty- to twenty-five-pound a month weight loss usually occurs only for the first month or two. After that an average of sixteen to eighteen pounds a month are lost. Even people who don't start off needing to lose many pounds can also expect the spectacular drop in the first month.

Are you startled by my telling you it will take months to take off your excess weight? Does it seem cruel and inhuman? Think about how many years it took you to put that weight on. Besides, a few months are really nothing as compared to the difference a normal weight will mean in the years to came.

Different people react differently to the program. Some people have no problems at all. The few that do have only minor, annoying "side effects" at the start of the fast. These are usually psychological.

A few complain that they are tired. Others will get minor headaches. Some might flirt briefly with vertigo or dizziness at a quick turn of the head. But rarely do these "side effects" last beyond the first week.

Your body has a much easier time accepting the regimen than your head does. Your mind just doesn't want to follow the game plan. It is comfortable with your old habits and will set up some papier-mâché roadblocks.

Drive right through.

Two of the few really physical reactions at the beginning might be diarrhea and minor nausea. The diarrhea is easily taken care of, with any number of products on the market your doctor may prescribe.

The nausea too can be easily dealt with, though it is not necessarily a bad side effect. It can work in your favor. After all, even your head won't want to eat if you're feeling a tinge of queaziness.

One word of caution. Be prepared to make frequent trips to the bathroom to urinate. After the first twenty-four hours, as I mentioned, the carbohydrate stores are eliminated. Carbohydrates tend to "dam" and sodium is released in a flood.

In the first week you have to fill out certain other forms that will help later in the restructuring of your eating attitudes.

One is a dietary history. It's a questionnaire asking what types of diets you've been on; where you eat meals away from home; the types of dietary supplements you may be taking; a typical prefasting eating day; where you get information on nutrition (advertising, books, magazines), etc.

There is also a psychological profile.


These first few days are the hump. Your difficulty will be in adjusting to any social and psychological annoyance that might arise rather than to anything physical. Your body is being well taken care of. The question is, what do you do with those extra hours? Food—thinking about meals, preparing meals, eating them—takes up a lot of time. In our society, eating is an ultrasocial phenomenon.

You have to shift your life orbit away from food. You have to turn your head around, look away from feasting to fasting.

After these first few days it gets easier. Losing weight,

you will recognize—because you have to—is far more important than the transitory gratification of eating.

REPEAT: This is cold turkey. There's no slow start, no coasting downhill to gain momentum. You go in from Day One and do it. The first few days may seem somewhat difficult because your head makes them that way. It's not hard for your body. There is no hunger, no physical need for food. The pounds disappear. And having them go with a minimum of psychic and almost no physical pain is incentive enough to continue, despite any minor psychological St. Vitus's Dance.

# 11

## *Prolinn*

IT's NOT as thick as Jell-O, but it doesn't run like water. It has the full-pink tint of a Beaujolais, but even the most uneducated of wine drinkers would not be fooled. It contains no fats, no carbohydrates, only a few calories, and an abundance of protein.

And it's what you will be substituting for the sustenance you're used to. It will provide your body with all the protein it needs. I call it Prolinn.

Nontechnically speaking, the formula is protein extracted from beef hides, concentrated into a palatable liquid form—palatable because it is heavily laced with a cherry flavoring. Without the flavoring, pure protein could be catalogued among the vilest and worst-tasting substances this side of Mercury.

The formula is composed of twenty of the twenty-two

amino acids, including all of the eight essential ones. It is predigested protein, predigested in that it has already been broken down into small peptides and amino acids. Here is a technical breakdown of Prolinn:

## PROLINN

NUTRITION INFORMATION:

| | | | |
|---|---|---|---|
| Calories | | Fats | 0 |
| (2 tablespoonfuls) | 60 | | |
| Protein | | Carbohydrates | 0 |
| (2 tablespoonsfuls) | 15 gm. | | |

AMINO ACIDS: Each 30m 1. (2 tablespoonfuls) provide approximately

| | | | |
|---|---|---|---|
| L-Alanine | 1300 mg. | L-Leucine | 450 mg. |
| L-Argine | 1200 mg. | L-Lysine | 650 mg. |
| L-Aspartic Acid | 900 mg. | L-Methionine | 110 mg. |
| L-Cystine | 10 mg. | L-Phenylananine | 350 mg. |
| L-Glutamic Acid | 1500 mg. | L-Proline | 2300 mg. |
| Glycine | 3500 mg. | L-Serine | 1000 mg. |
| L-Histidine | 110 mg. | L-Threonine | 300 mg. |
| L-Hydroxylysine | 150 mg. | L-Tryptophane | 65 mg. |
| L-Hydroxyproline | 1000 mg. | L-Tyrosine | 100 mg. |
| L-Isoleucine | 200 mg. | L-Valine | 350 mg. |

SOLUBLE PROTEIN HYDROLYSATE . . . . . . . . . . . . 15 GM. PER 30 ML.

This formula is necessary for the program to work properly. It allows you to lose as much as thirty pounds of fat safely in a single month.

Prolinn is what will keep you in nitrogen balance so you don't suffer a fast weight gain once you start eating again.

Expect to be full of energy and bounce, clearer thinking and better feeling than you've been in years—or perhaps ever before. Your own body and mental attitude are doing this for you.

Prolinn is one of the best protein sources discovered up to this time. Previously it was believed that albumin —egg whites—was the uppermost limit, the most complete protein.

One study compared the Prolinn formula with meat and fish and found that the formula resulted in a similar protein level as meat. Another study found the same to be true comparing the formula to egg whites.

There is no such thing as a completely pure food. Meat, fish and eggs will have some fat. By taking Prolinn, the guesswork is gone, no measuring or weighing of food is needed. We know exactly what you are getting and how much you are getting. You are getting what your body needs—protein.

If you're expecting Prolinn to taste like an ice cream soda, you're in for a disappointment. Although it's not as bad tasting as some medicines can be (some patients actually like it), it may be easier for you to think of Prolinn as medicine. Obesity is as much a disease as pneumonia or swine flu. You want to be cured. You're going to cure yourself and Prolinn is going to assist you.

We are trying to break your eating habits. Prolinn should not be thought of as gratification, as you've always thought of your food. However, most fasters do get to like the taste of Prolinn and look forward to their daily allotment.

Some drink it straight. Others mix it with water or club soda. But remember—it isn't food, certainly not as you've been conditioned to think of food. The formula is part of a medical program that will leave you thin.

Prolinn will be the assist that will help you to lose fat weight and gain good health. That and your own determination.

# 12

## *Psychology of Fasting*

A PEANUT. Maybe a pizza. A Nutty Coconut ice cream cone or the most sumptuous five-course meal in the best French restaurant.

It might have been almost anything that pushed you "off the wagon" in the past. Any little bit of food that you rationalized, "Well, just this one thing won't hurt." And then, depressed and angry with yourself, you start eating again. And your diet goes down the garbage disposal.

On this fast there are no temptations, no little inch to give yourself. What you "eat" has already been decided upon. What goes into your mouth is predetermined.

You have no decisions to make. And losing weight is going to be much easier for you than it has ever been before.

There is no prescribed exercise connected with the protein-sparing fast program. However, there is one exercise that I would like you to do. Fill a carton or a suitcase with the heaviest things available, until the scale accurately reflects the number of pounds you know that you are overweight.

Pick it up. Pick it up if you can! Now think about the fact that this heavy burden—this sack of extra poundage—is what you're carrying around in your body *every second of every minute of every hour of every day!*

If the pounds are too many for you to pick up without risking a rupture, can you imagine what a strain you are putting on your heart?! Try taking a five-pound sack of sugar or ten pounds of potatoes and carrying them around with you for an entire day!

Do you wonder why you will feel so magnificently wonderful after the first week, when you will have certainly shed the first six to ten pounds?

She loves clothes and now she can be fashionably dressed.

Gay W. is in her forties and has four teenaged daughters. Though not a member of the jet set, she is nevertheless financially well off, with a husband who often takes her flying to Europe. He could eat all those heavily-sauced creations of the French kitchens without their becoming a permanent part of his anatomy, but Gay had "been like a yoyo most of the time."

Weight went on easily and came off hard. She even endured the rice diet at Duke University—got a little slimmer, but soon was a heavyweight again. "I think it was Christmas that blew it that time."

Gay lost thirty pounds in her first five weeks with me, eighty pounds altogether. She can now slink in clinging clothes with the best of them and not look like a pregnant hippopotamus in the blowsy peasant look.

"This fast works partly because you do see results so rapidly, but also because if you eat, each bite of food is a stimulus. For anyone who loves to eat, it's like trying to eat just one peanut. Try to get someone who loves sweets to eat one bite of lemon meringue pie. You can't do it. It's better to say no to it."

Granted, rationally deciding not to eat for however long it takes would seem to require a certain amount of masochism. The fact is the opposite: finally you're being very good to yourself! In the past you were programmed, habituated and seduced into eating. Television tantalizes you with crackling corn chips, gurgling mountain-stream-cold beer, candy bars, cakes, little tiny circles of spaghetti—and that's just for commercial openers.

Radio expounds the "ultimate pleasure" of eating. Glossy magazines display perfectly decorated, excruciatingly appetizing food layouts. Sides of buses exhort you to nibble on cake that's tastee or to buy a special-recipe bread. It's all around you, teasing you, reminding you—and, yes, a certain degree of masochism is needed to turn your stomach away from eating.

But it's not forever. You are merely postponing eating your food—postponing eating until the time you are slim and able to enjoy foods that won't ever let you become fat again.

Don't ever try to understand why people try to sabotage you. It happens all the time and it happens to almost everyone.

' Husbands who always said they wanted their wives thin again suddenly become uncomfortable as the weight goes and the attractiveness grows. "You've lost enough," they'll say. "You look fine now."

"Just have something to eat."

It's almost a plea.

"Just have something. Eat a little something."

This is the most repeated advice you will hear from others who somehow can't adjust to what you're doing.

"You'll kill yourself," some will go so far as to say. They've suddenly become weight specialists!

Ridiculous.

Many of my patients are so thin-oriented that they host fabulous dinners at fabulous restaurants, all the while limiting their own feasting to a diet soda, a club soda, or ice water. For dessert they treat themselves to two sticks of sugar-free chewing gum.

Ignore the plaintive wails, the expressions of anxiety and the sugar-coated, poison-filled words of advice.

If the onslaught upsets you, avoid going to restaurants. But if you have half a sense of humor, you can laugh off all of the idle chatter and get-fat-again forgeries that pass for friendly advice.

The only advice worth taking: don't try to please everyone. Please yourself. Be for you first.

I can't tell you how many times I have patients—most often women—who will blame someone else for their cheating.

"It's my husband's fault," the refrain goes. "I went off the program because he threatened me. He said he had this function, this social event, this banquet, and if I don't eat, he'll divorce me."

You have to learn to be assertive. Don't cop-out. Don't let other people bully you into harming yourself. You have to tell people that you're doing something you must do and that they shouldn't be bothered by it.

Assert yourself for yourself.


Barbara's mother was appalled when she came home from college for Christmas break. Her daughter had been heavy since she was a toddler—but now she was close to elephantine.

Barbara couldn't remember the last time she had had

a date—she had long since given up going to the mixers. Her favorite night of the week was Sunday, when the dorm cafeteria was shut down and the girls on her floor trooped off to a pizza place where Barbara loved to overindulge. Weighing in at 192, Barbara was sixty-two pounds overweight. That's all past-tense. Today she's a slim 130 pounds and looks as good as any homecoming queen.

"When I first heard about your program," she told me, "I told myself 'I can't do that, it's much too drastic.' But I was in drastic shape.

"Once on the program, I got used to not eating. At first I couldn't stand to be around food. Then after a couple of weeks, I could read recipes and help in the kitchen. The smell of food didn't bother me."

It doesn't take long to fall into the pattern of the fast, to start accepting emotionally the path you've rationally decided to follow. You do get used to the notion. Where food had once been your major daily "reward," your new gratification is that climb onto the scale each morning. Your reward is those pounds that once were yours, but are not anymore.

Before long, you may begin to find that's it's not *your* head that needs adjusting, it's those around you.

At first, you might feel uneasy at parties or dinner parties. "If someone came to my house and refused to eat," you might rationalize," "I would be offended. I'd better not go to so-and-so's party. She might be offended."

But there is nothing to be offended by. You are curing a disease. You are under treatment and making yourself better. Any friend should be able to understand that and wish you well.

But, nonetheless, some do get uneasy. Other people can't handle your fasting, although you can.

Larry G. is a forty-six-year-old widower. He was not overly heavy when he started the program, but he had to lose—desperately.

Larry has a heart condition. He already has suffered one coronary.

When his wife died, he realized that those extra pounds could very likely leave his two daughters completely alone in the world. Now that they had only one parent, Larry wanted to give himself a better chance of sticking around to raise them.

Larry's motivation was so overwhelmingly strong, he didn't waste any time creating psychological problems for himself. But he found that his dinner partners had a much more difficult time adjusting.

"Psychologically, it bothered them more than it bothered me. Their attitude was "I can't eat if you're not eating.""

But that's their problem. You're the one carrying the extra baggage on your body, not them. You're the one increasing your chances of a heart attack, early diabetes, gall stones—not them. And it's you who soon will be able to zipper your trousers without a struggle or keep your blouse buttoned. It will be you who will be modeling a new silhouette.

You're almost there. You've lost eighty percent of the weight you needed to. The protein-sparing fast will soon be at an end. You'll start eating solid food again.

Beware! This is a stage in your life fraught with peril! Your doctor may be needed to keep you in the right direction.

Some patients need reminding at this point that they committed themselves to go down—all the way. If someone has cancer, it does no good to cut out ninety-five percent of the tumor. The entire mass should be expunged or you face the very real probability of its growing again.

Because of those metabolic changes that occur in the fat person, you should go all the way. You must bring your metabolism back into the proper balance or fall victim to those vicious fat cycles. The first secret for maintaining your newly-won weight loss is to get down to a normal poundage.

It is great when a patient loses sixty pounds—but if

he needs to lose a hundred, it's not great enough. If twenty-five was the goal, twenty doesn't cut it.

Those last few pounds may be the toughest—and not just because of you.

You must be careful of the well-meaning husband, wife, or friend, probably both flabbergasted and delighted with your loss, who counsels that you've "lost enough and don't need to lose anymore."

Sometimes they will even start saying that you're too skinny and won't look good if you lose more.

It's likely they are not accustomed to seeing you slim. They're used to the fat you and haven't adjusted to the new thin you.

But this problem is a tiny blemish, a pimple that barely breaks the surface and will soon disappear. Just admire yourself in the mirror and love the image you see. And keep on the program until your doctor says you're finished.

REPEAT: If you're like most protein-sparing fasters, this will be the easiest dieting program you've ever tried, because there are no temptations and no decisions. Give yourself that self-injection of firm resolve to start the program. The results will be well worth it. You're going to love yourself again.

# 13

## *Motivation*

I F YOU'RE LIKE most overweight people, you've done a lot of thinking about why you'd like to lose weight and the advantages of being thinner.

You've got to really want to lose weight, but wishing won't make it happen. You've got to be motivated. And that has to come from you. Once you decide that you really want to lose your extra pounds, my program is going to help you do it—really do it this time.

You may already know your reasons for wanting to be slim, but here are some reminders of why you should start the protein-sparing fast program now.

### 1.
You've tried everything else—and everything else has failed.

2.

It's new. Going back to old diets—even when they worked once—is an odds-against-you proposition.

3.

Unlike other diets and quite different from fad approaches, getting weight off is not the goal. The behavior modification will help you to keep it off. *That's* the goal.

4.

You owe it to yourself to become slim again (or for the first time in your life) so that you can feel good.

5.

Slimming down will slim down the chances of your developing any one of a number of obesity-related diseases.

6.

You're going to look better. This isn't going to revolutionize your social life, but it will alter and enhance your own self-image and help you to make peace with yourself.

7.

This fast frees you from having to cut, measure and weigh. You have no further food decisions to make until you've reached your desired weight.

8.

With the protein-sparing fast program, once you take it off, the chances are excellent that you'll keep it off.

9.

Once committed, you can cook for others or sit with others while they feast and it will not shake your resolve or divert you from your path.

10.

You will be giving your body a rest from any personal food allergens you may have . . . and as your system is cleansed you will probably feel better than you've felt in years.

11.

You don't count calories and so you don't have to barter with yourself or fight temptation.

12.

There are no drugs or medications involved in this healthful approach to the new (permanently new!) you.

13.

It's safe: there has not been a reported case of any permanent bad effects although thousands of patients have completed the fast successfully.

14.

You don't fight hunger—as you invariably do on 1,000 or 1,500 calorie diets.

15.

It's the quickest way to lose weight.

16.

It's a can't-fail approach: you can actually chart your own weight loss.

*17.*

It's excuse-free. You can carry your Prolinn anywhere. It requires no special preparation and does not spoil in normal heat or cold weather.

*18.*

Instead of being tired, you will often find that you have more natural energy than you know what to do with!

*19.*

It is the single approach that has found nothing but support among top medical men.

*20.*

Safe—quick—sure—and the one approach that will work just when you've about given up hope of ever shedding that extra weight again.

*21.*

Your weight loss will be so immediate and so astonishing that your own scale will give you constant reinforcement and enthusiasm.

*22.*

Losing your extra weight on my protein-sparing fast program will let you live a longer life . . .

*23.*

. . . and enjoy every moment of it.

# 14

## What Ifs

WHAT IF YOU'VE decided this is it—your last chance? You have to lose weight. You're tired of being fat and miserable. This is it. The motivation is there and you want to begin my protein-sparing fast program.

But—a terrible word in the dieter's vocabulary—what if you have this trip to Europe planned that you've saved for for the last five years. You've already paid the travel agent. There's no backing out. Besides, your husband, wife or best friend would be disappointed. What if you *just* can't be on the Prolinn formula for those two weeks?

Should you put off beginning the fast? Wait until you get back?

No.

Your self-motivation is high, it's not the time to change your mind.

Exceptions can be made under special rare circumstances. I have had patients who've gone on cruises where for two weeks extravagant meals were the chief entertainment, and these patients have stuck to their Prolinn regimen.

But I have had other patients where interruptions couldn't be helped.

In these rare cases, I will have the patient switch from the Prolinn to baked or broiled lean meat and fish. The patient will eat seven to eight ounces a day of lean meat and fish instead of the Prolinn. Although meat is not as efficient as the formula, for a short period of time it will not be detrimental to the fast. The patient will stay in ketosis (alleviating hunger) and can ease back into the regular program on his return.

This is not recommended, but it's not disastrous.

What would be disastrous is putting off your weight loss until tomorrow. By tomorrow you can have already lost two, three, four pounds!

# 15

## *Fringe Benefits of the Protein-Sparing Fast*

THE MAJOR BENEFITS of the protein-sparing fast program are obvious. By losing your weight and keeping it off, you reduce your chance of heart disease. It decreases the likelihood and may very well prevent the onset of diabetes.

The lost weight reduces your blood pressure.

People with bad backs or poor knees or some other structural defect take that extra pressure off already insulted parts of their bodies.

But there is one benefit that might not be so obvious to you, and it has to do with your allergies.


When most people think of allergies, they think of hives from strawberries or reactions to medication.

149

But most of us actually have reactions to other foods that we do not ordinarily associate as allergic symptoms. Some of the symptoms of these allergies may be:

| | |
|---|---|
| *nervousness* | *abnormal tiredness* |
| *dizziness* | *indigestion* |
| *constipation* | *neuralgia* |
| *canker sores* | *sinusitis* |
| *heartburn* | *hypertension* |
| *migraines* | *hemorrhoids* |
| *epilepsy* | *chest pains* |
| *irritability* | |

Often doctors will misdiagnose allergies. One fringe benefit of my fast is that by not eating, you are eliminating all your food allergens. The symptoms of the allergies then clear up spontaneously.

When allergic symptoms in the refeeding period reappear I send some of my patients to a doctor specializing in food allergies for a testing with a new technique. When the food villains are isolated, you are able to eliminate them from your diet or, in some cases the doctor can make up a liquid that, when placed under your tongue, will allow you to eat the food allergen without reacting to it on a one-shot basis.

# 16

## Side Effects

*"I feel great. I'm amazed. I went through the stupid routine of going on pills. I thought the weight loss justified the side effects. But if anyone told me fasting would make me feel so good with absolutely no side effects, I wouldn't have believed them."*

—A thirty-eight-year-old patient, who lost eighty-eight pounds.

H ARD TO BELIEVE? Protein-sparing fasting might appear to some people to be such a drastic, extreme measure that your body would have to react to in some detrimental way.

That's what it might seem.

But that isn't the case at all.

*There are no major side effects on the Last Chance Diet program.*

There may be some minor ones, but they are strictly minor and not difficult to overcome. At worst they are inconveniences. And, at worst, only a few people will experience them. You might very likely feel nothing but

153

exhilaration and well-being—and pride as your waistline gets smaller.

The minor side effects—hardly more than annoyances—range from a lightheadedness to diarrhea.

They include:

*Slight intolerance to cold.*

*Dry skin.*

*Hair loss.* Approximately five percent of my patients will notice they are losing some hair. Usually they are the only ones who notice the difference. Nobody else does. This loss is only temporary and minimal, and the hair grows back after the fast.

*Fatigue.* Some patients complain of fatigue during the first week. Generally it is a psychological state rather than a physical one. They are actually depressed that their food has been taken away. All that's needed is a short adjustment period. Unless, of course, we uncover some metabolic problem.

*Bad breath.* This is by far the most common side effect. Ketosis can cause halitosis. But mouthwashes and breath drops minimize this problem.

*Cramps in the extremities.* Toe cramps or finger cramps bother a very, very few patients. The doctor needs only to increase their calcium supplement, and the cramps go away.

*Nausea.* Some people react to the production of ketones, and have a slight degree of nausea. The nausea very rarely lasts and can be treated.

*Gas.* This is one of the more difficult problems to deal with. But compared to the weight loss and how you feel otherwise, it's a small annoyance to have to put up with.

Women may find that their menstrual cycle is altered. They may have spotting. Their period may come early, late or might be exceptionally heavy. It may happen, but is no cause for any great concern.

According to Alvin F. Goldfarb, M.D., clinical professor of obstetrics and gynecology at the University of Pennsylvania's School of Medicine, whenever a woman's nutrition is markedly altered her menstrual cycle is likely to change. It is not only the protein-sparing fast that would cause these deviations, but other diets as well. Change her nutritional pattern, and the cycle will behave differently.

These are all minor. There are no major side effects.

No changes in the blood composition.

No kidney complications.

No liver complications.

Cuts and wounds heal normally.

In short, you are able to maintain your life style with only slight modifications, knowing that you will not start to feel run down. Should you experience any side effects, discuss them with your doctor. He can recommend additional vitamin or mineral supplements. He can prescribe something to clear up any diarrhea or to keep your skin from drying out. Follow his directions.

One question that everyone who hears about the fast asks—even the most delicate people!—concerns your bowel movements. I often get perturbed patients, worried because they haven't moved their bowels in days.

Naturally some fasters may go for five to six days without a movement. It is nothing to worry about. Sometimes a patient will complain of constipation, almost out of reflex. He believes he should be constipated because he hasn't had a bowel movement. Sometimes a laxative is necessary, but not often. Or you can take a weekly enema. But most of my patients move their bowels every other day, some daily. Your doctor will advise you.

REPEAT: Rest assured that the protein-sparing fast has *no* major side effects. What minor ones that might occur are far fewer and often easier to cope with than those on many other less "extreme" diet regimens.

# 17

*Plateaus*

*"Plateaus? Never hit one. My weight loss*
*was one steady linear curve*
*from start to finish."*

—A fifty-two-year-old male patient
who lost more than fifty pounds.

P LATEAUS ARE POSSIBLE, even on my program. But they
are much more common on other diets and regimens.

Plateaus are those demoralizing humps that have probably accounted for more people falling off the dieting wagon than all the Sara Lee banana cakes ever baked.

A pound lost. Another pound gone. You're elated. Until one day the scale doesn't budge. You've stopped losing. And the next day, the scale still doesn't budge. You become discouraged, disgusted, and wonder what went wrong.

"Why am I torturing myself cutting calories/carbohydrates/eating just grapefruit/stuffing myself with bananas/whatever diet you were on—for nothing?" you ask just before plunging into an eating binge. Once again, a plateau has assassinated your will power, a delicate object at best.

I did say that plateaus can occur on my program. They are possible. But most of my patients, like the one quoted earlier, *never hit them.* They lose steadily, without interruption.

However, there are times, for some people, that the scale marker holds to a fixed spot for anywhere from two to seven days.

It's a discouragement—*but not a disaster.* (The disaster would be if you used this as an excuse to give up.) You must remember that it is the scale that is not moving. A scale is nothing more than a piece of metal. It has no ability to interpret what kind of weight it is measuring. If you put a bucket filled with ten pounds of water or one with ten pounds of fat on a scale, the reading will be ten pounds. The scale can only register a number. But, there is a vast difference between the amounts of fat, water, muscle, bone that you carry.

A scale is often the worst "friend" a dieter can have. When your weight is the same, or perhaps even a pound more than the day before, your inclination might be to depress yourself by telling yourself "I'm not losing" or "I've gained a pound of fat."

*The probability is that neither statement is true.*

There are reasons why some people hit plateaus that have nothing to do with losing or not losing fat.

You must not overlook the basic concept of the protein-sparing fast and energy consumption.

Your body has to have energy to function. It takes energy to breathe, sleep, watch television, add a string of numbers or compete in the Olympic Decathalon. If the only source of energy is from within your body, that's where the fuel has to come from.

When you're on this fast, your primary source of energy is your fat. You've lived a day, that means you've used energy that day. Some of your fat store has got to have been depleted—whether or not your scale mirrors that fact.

Don't be addicted to your scale. It is a beneficial instrument as long as it doesn't discourage you.

You musn't forget that that pesky pointer might stop at the same number, your overall weight might be the same, but your *body size* is diminishing. It has to.

The real test of whether you're still losing *fat* is not the scale, but the acetone levels on your breath. This is even more accurate than urinary ketones. There is a machine that can test this level. Even if your scale weight stays the same, we can tell you are still losing fat, with this piece of medical equipment.

There are several possibilities why you might plateau. Women are far more likely to do so than men, female hormones being the chief culprit. These hormones cause a woman to retain water much more easily than a man does. At times there is virtually "water intoxication."

Water retention (medical term: *edema*) is no reason to cut down on the amount of fluid you drink. On the contrary, water itself is a natural diuretic. But it may be advisable, if a plateau is hit, to reduce the number of bottles of diet soda you drink. Although they are sugarless and free of carbohydrates, diet sodas do contain a trace of sodium—which promotes water retention. (One of my patients estimated that he was spending thirty dollars a week on diet sodas. But he, like so many others, had no problems with hitting a loss hump.)

(The money spent on diet sodas isn't all "extra expense" inasmuch as you are saving lots of dollars on your food bill.)

Body water is also produced from oxidation. Water is a by-product of the oxidation of triglycerides. You will be using triglycerides as an energy source and occasionally fluid might build up.

This weight is fluid—you're not getting "heavier" in that you're not getting "fatter."

Again, there are far fewer and shorter plateaus on this program than others, but if you're one of the few unlucky ones to hit a plateau, don't let this psychological hazard deter you. You are losing fat and will continue to lose it. Keep your expectations focused on that monthly loss and not on a daily or weekly one.

Of course, there is another cause for plateaus—cheating.

Lynn lost thirteen pounds in two weeks, but then, at the beginning of the third, her weight was up a pound.

When I asked her if she knew why she gained, her answer was, "It's called horseradish sauce, I was making it and sampling it."

Once in a while you might cheat, but you're going to find that the temptation to do so is slight. On other diets, you're putting food into your mouth. There's always the enticement to put more in than you should or to put something in that you shouldn't at all. No such temptation on this program. More than likely, you won't cheat. If you do, don't hate yourself. It's easy enough to get back on the right track.

Cheating doesn't destroy your chances. It merely delays the happy day when you'll reach goal one.

Just keep in mind my patient who went from 209 pounds to 135, all the while cooking and shopping for her husband and twelve children.

REPEAT: Many people on the protein-sparing fast do not hit plateaus. Their weight-loss is a continual pound after pound drop. The few people who do hit plateaus get off them quickly. The important thing to remember is that a plateau is usually nothing more than water retention. Your body size is getting smaller even if your scale doesn't reflect it.

# 18

## Who Can't Fast

THE PROTEIN-SPARING fast isn't for everyone—but there are very few who can't go on it.

Surprisingly few. Doctors have even okayed the fast for certain cancer patients and patients with other debilitating diseases.

Basically, there are only four categories of people who should not start this program.

Pregnant women.

People with malfunctioning livers.

People with kidney failure.

People with certain types of heart diseases.

If you don't fall into any of those categories and need to lose twenty pounds or more, stop torturing yourself. Make a resolution. Start this program. You've got nothing to lose but your weight.

# 19

## *History of Fasting*

TOTAL FASTING is as old as man. Man has abstained from eating any food for protracted periods of time from his first sighting on the evolutionary tableau.

Early man, so the anthropologists tell us, was a hunter and forager. Not as strong or fleet as many of the competing hunters, he had to use guile and wile to make a kill.

But game wasn't always available, and when it was around, it sometimes declined man's invitation to dinner. No food meant man didn't eat. In fact, among the many theories is one that man turned eventually to husbandry to insure a steadier food source.

But total fasting at one time or another during the year remained part of man's life for three principal reasons—magic, ethics, and religion.

Primitive peoples who believed that objects and natural phenomena—rain storms, floods, the moon, the stars—were alive with a consciousness and a soul often believed that fasting could somehow influence these objects and phenomena. They used a fast to gain a magical hold over Nature and her frightening powers. You want more ears of corn this year? Don't eat and you get a magical edge on the Great Crop God, was the reasoning.

Medicine men and tribal priests would fast to encourage hallucinations and visions. Prolonged total fasting may bring on effects similar to a good jolt of LSD.

The Indians of North America thought that the long periods of fasting were a sure sign of power and endurance. Not ones to do things halfway, however, they went without water, too.

Total fasting has been an element of religions—primitive and modern.

Today, for example, Jews do not eat from sundown the day before to sundown the day of their holiday Yom Kippur. Various groups of Jews also have twelve-hour fasts on other days. At one point Catholics practiced a forty-day pre-Easter fast.

During their month of Ramadan, Muslims do not eat or drink as long as there is enough light to differentiate between a black thread and a white one.

Fasting was once a more integral part of western religion but after awhile it was decided that too much of it was overly weakening the worshippers. And weakened worshippers, it was thought, couldn't work as well and contribute as much to their God.

Total fasting has also been undertaken as a virtue, a show of moral character, or as a benefit to the community. Mahatma Gandhi went on many of his fasts as a protest against British rule.

The "purifying" nature of the fast, its "cleansing effect," its "purity" gave it an ethical nature.

Total fasting has been used as protest, too. In 1976, one Irish nationalist, trying to get transferred from a British prison to one in Northern Ireland, died after a 61-day period of no eating.

You will start your protein-sparing fast for none of these reasons. Your fasting is for one reason, and one reason only.

It's for you.

A healthier you.

# 20

## *Dangers of Total Fasting*

TOTAL FASTING has been promoted recently as the "Ultimate Diet," the diet to end all diets. Tragically, that is exactly what it was for one twenty-year-old English woman.

This particular total faster stopped eating altogether for thirty weeks. She managed to lose more than one hundred pounds—along with her life.

Nine days after she resumed eating, the woman died. An autopsy revealed that in those weeks of total fasting, she had used up more than half of her lean body mass—including part of her heart.

Death from total fasting can occur in other ways besides "myocardial atrophy" — this destruction of the heart.

There have been cases where the kidneys of a total

177

faster have stopped functioning, causing death. In other instances, a total faster's heart has failed when he or she has taken a water pill.

Extensive medical supervision is necessary if total fasting is to last longer than a week. There are silent problems that can develop—problems of which the patients are unaware. If a total fast is to go on for any length of time, I concur with the top medical experts in the field who advocate hospitalization. Even then, however, all the dangers are not removed. Even with hospitalization, total fasting is not a recommended program.

Total fasting is a serious, dangerous method of losing weight. It throws your body out of "balance" and can create some serious conditions—one being an inflammation of the nerves. A total faster may find that nerves in various parts of his body, especially his arms and legs, are pulsing with pain.

Total fasting may lead to anemia. Lab test reports of a total faster can often be abnormal. Specific liver function tests may be abnormal. So too many reports on kidney function tests.

The total faster may find that his body has trouble using vitamin B, potassium, and sodium.

In one case a patient on a total fast died by "drowning" in his own fluids. This person had not been excreting enough sodium. Sodium encourages water retention leading to too much fluid in the person's body—and in this case eventually leading to his demise.

With all these dangers, the clear fact is that total fasting does not accomplish your goal—does not give you the weight loss commensurate with the jeopardy in which you place yourself.

Again, I repeat, only half the weight you lose on a total fast within the first couple of months is what you want to lose—fat. The rest is lean body tissue. You are destroying your energy-using potential, making it even harder for you to lose weight. The less muscle you have, the less energy you can expend. And so we return to the equation that energy is food and fat is stored excess energy.

Unlike the protein-sparing fast where you're not depleting your muscles and protein-store, on a total fast you are subject to considerable fatigue and a loss of stamina. You will tire easily and find it harder and harder to keep up your normal pace. A study at the University of California found that patients under observation on a total fast began to have irregular heartbeats whenever they exercised.

This is not so on my program. The energy you may feel, the all-round sense of well-being is not a false condition. Your body is not being deprived of what it needs to function efficiently and well. You are in proper "balance" and will remain so throughout the fast.

Total fasting can also send the dieter into a psychological tailspin since a resumption of eating brings on a rapid weight gain. Your body is compelled to replace the lost muscle and protein tissue and convert any food it gets into lean body tisue. You can very easily put on fifteen pounds within days after you start to eat again. A weight gain after a long period of self-control and discipline is enough to send anyone into the depths of dieter's depression.

REPEAT: Total fasting is a potentially dangerous and harmful way of losing weight. Ill effects from a total fast can range from constant pain and unfavorable and acute biochemical changes to death. What is more, weight lost on a total fast in the first month or so is not the weight you want to lose. Only fifty per cent of it is fat, the rest is lean body tissue. A resumption of eating brings on a rapid weight return.

# 21

# Games Your Doctor Might Play

Lorry, with her pixie-tousled hair and freckled face, looked more like a high school freshman than the fulltime bookkeeper and mother of three she was. And she had a figure that would have looked right at home in a stadium leading rahs and sis-boom-bahs.

She had been on my program for four months and was ecstatic with her sixty-six-pound weight loss. It was her last visit. She had accomplished what she had come to do—lose weight. Now she was confident that the job and, family tensions were no longer going to be "solved" in the refrigerator. She had her weight off and she knew she wasn't going to be a fatty again.

But Lorry had one last thing to say to me.

"Doctor Linn," she began. "I wasn't sure I was going to make it through the program when I first started.

And it was all because of one stupid little thing—I hate waiting. And you always had me waiting.

"But after a while, it didn't bother me at all. I looked forward to talking to the other patients. Telling them how I was doing. Getting encouragement the couple of times I hit a plateau. And then I figured it out—you made us wait on purpose, so we would talk."

She was right. Sitting for an extra couple of minutes before seeing one of the staff is an excellent form of supportive therapy. When you're doing well, boasting gives you a boost. And if you're not doing as well as you might have hoped, listening to other patients tell of their progress helps you, too.

Very often people don't have a very good self body image. They look into the mirror, but they don't really see themselves. Or as one patient expressed it, "It took me a long time to believe my friends when they said I was looking slimmer. I knew what the scale read—I knew I was getting lighter, but I still thought of myself as a fatty."

But if you can't see yourself, you can see other people. You see them week after week and the change in them is startling. One woman who lost fifty-three pounds complained that she never saw the same people from visit to visit, until it dawned on her that she did, but she didn't recognize them!

# 22

## Twenty Questions

S o far i have avoided burdening you with medical references and scientific jargon. You aren't here for a medical education, so I have talked to you in clear simple language.

It is often sad to listen to the ignorance of basic nutrition truths expressed by the men and women who come to see me for the first time.

They ask a lot of questions, and that's good. It indicates that they're searching for answers.

Here are twenty of the most often asked questions. In a few cases I have used medical terminology in the answers—but not enough to cloud your understanding.

You may have other questions. The physician who will supervise your protein-sparing fast can answer them. Don't be shy about asking.

*1. Is there any real difference in the food habits of people who are overweight and people who are not other than the quantities of food consumed?*

Yes. The U.S. Public Health Service confirms my own findings when they report that "The one general difference in this country between the food habits of the people who are or are not obese is that the obese tend to overeat in the evening."

Time and time again I have listened to patients explain how they "watch themselves" at meals but somehow don't consider nighttime snacking as "really eating." It "doesn't really seem to count."

*2. That being the case, would it help to put a lock on the refrigerator or to keep away from it altogether?*

The behavior modification part of my program will train you on where to eat, when to eat, and how to eat. Incidentally, the refrigerator is not the biggest enemy of most overweights. Snack foods—candies and cookies and cakes—are not kept in refrigerators.

*3. I have always watched my diet and eaten only the right foods: healthful foods. How could I have gotten fat?*

Many people misunderstand why they are fat. They pay attention to what they eat but ignore quantities. It will not hurt you to become aware of the caloric content of some of those very nourishing foods. You'll understand why one glass of milk may be okay but four glasses add up to mucho added fat reserves.

*4. Are women fatter than men?*

Yes. Fat comprises a higher percentage of total body weight in the female than in the male. However in adult life body fat increases at a faster rate for men than for women.

For women, excessive weight gain occurs more frequently after age twenty, during pregnancy, and after menopause. Men tend to gain weight between twenty-five and 40 years of age.

5. *Do men lose weight more quickly than women?*

Very often. The explanation is a complicated one, but you can be assured that if you are a woman and stick with it, you'll lose all the weight you want to lose —though it may take you a few weeks longer than your male counterpart.

6. *Can an overweight person be undernourished?*

Absolutely. That excess poundage is not necessarily a storehouse of nutritional reserves. You may actually be overweight and badly undernourished. Some vitamins cannot be stored by the body at all. If you take in more of these vitamins than your body needs on any given day, they will be excreted.

7. *Fatness runs in my family. Does this make my case hopeless?*

Studies show that obesity may be the result of both genetic and environmental factors. Seven out of every ten patients I treat report that one or both of their parents were overweight.

If your mother and/or father were/are fat, you have a greater chance of becoming fat yourself. But *you* did

it to yourself. Nobody held your mouth open and forci-
bly fed you all those excess calories. By the same rule,
you can make yourself thin and stay thin.

8. *I am in good health except for my overweight.*
*Does this still mean that I have a more likely chance of*
*dying earlier than I would if I were thin?*

I'm afraid so.

There is no doubt that the overweight and mortality
relationship is real. And incidentally, it's time you got
thin *once and for all.* Being overweight is dangerous.
You add to the dangers when you fad-diet your way
down and up and down and up.

Want more bad news? Cardiac enlargement and
heart failure are often directly attributable to obesity.

Pretty lady, you should know that obesity increases
your risk of skin ulcers.

Arthritis sufferers must face up to the knowledge that
obesity often compounds the physical immobilization
that accompanies arthritis.

9. *Are diuretics recommended for diets? How about*
*appetite depressant pills?*

According to the U.S. Public Health Service, the
routine use of diuretics in weight-reducing, regimens is
unlikely to be of any value. Their sustained use can
cause renal damage.

Most appetite-depressant drugs are sympath-omime-
tic amines related in structure to amphetamine. In most
cases, after about 6 weeks of use, the amphetamines
cease to have their original effect of diminishing appetite. Insomnia, irritability, restlessness, tenseness,

sweating, dry mouth, and alterations in the gastrointestinal function are the reported side effects.

"Adrenergic effects on the cardiovascular system make the use of anorexigenic agents especially hazardous for patients with cardiac disease."

*10. How do I know your program isn't just another fad diet?*

Fad diets may have a short-term effect but the weight loss, when you win it, comes and goes in a minute. They have little lasting or practical value.

It is important when taking off pounds that you are nutritionally sound and not hungry. This program fills both of those needs.

I cannot tell you often enough that taking your weight off is not the goal. Follow the program and I can assure you the weight will come off. The goal is to keep it off. That's why I cannot stress too much the importance of the refeeding period and the behavior modification training.

*11. If I'm "good" and am true to your program for a few weeks, would it then be okay to break it up with something simple like a salad?*

No. Sorry. But in a couple of weeks a salad will seem like a sirloin steak to you, and in a couple of months it will seem like strawberry shortcake. There are both psychological and physiological reasons why you shouldn't. For one thing, it may take you out of ketosis and that could delay your reaching your desired weight by three or four days.

*12. But what if I do? What if I "fall off the wagon?"*

As psychologist Dr. Albert Ellis would say, "Tough shit." And then he cautions you not to hate yourself or become guilt ridden. What you do is start again—not tomorrow or next Monday but this minute.

In the old days of diet-failure, do you remember how often you would set New Year's Day or the first of the month or "Next Monday" as the beginning again? Not with me. Not with this program. You begin again *now*. Instantly.

*13. But you're taking away all of my food? Isn't that too drastic?*

I'm offering you good health, good appearance, and lots of added self-esteem in return. And it isn't nearly as drastic as those artificial approaches such as the by-pass operations and the people who have their jaw wired together.

*14. How about if I just chew some food and spit it out and rinse my mouth and brush my teeth so nothing goes down?*

How about recognizing that no matter how carefully you think you are about it, something is going to be ingested. Instead, reach for a stick of Trident or Carefree or some other brand of sugarless chewing gum. They even have sugar-free bubble gum.

*15. Won't I feel strange not eating when people around me are eating?*

You'll feel any way you tell yourself you feel. To paraphrase Dr. Ellis again, most of how we feel comes from the words we tell ourselves. I know one patient who said he began to feel like a visitor from another planet. He saw the food commercials on TV and the people eating snack foods in the street and realized that he had no relation to it. "It was," he said, "as if it were all turtle food or fish food."

*16. If you've told me to take eight ounces of Prolinn a day and I only take six, will that speed my weight loss?*

Don't do it. The extra two ounces amount to fewer than 120 calories. The Prolinn is needed in ample enough quantity to fill your need for a nitrogen balance.

*17. Is it okay if I help myself with mental crutches?*

Sure. But don't help yourself with drugs or stimulants unless I or your supervising physician prescribes them. I know one person who was having attitude problems until he realized that all of that costly restaurant food he had filled himself with eventually turned to excretion. Whenever he found himself fighting temptation, he imagined the desired food object as excretion. Needless to say, it killed all desire to deviate from the program!

*18. I'm worried that when I get my weight down I will put it on again. I'm literally afraid to begin eating again.*

As often as not, you will continue to lose weight on my refeeding program. Your anxiety is natural and only experience will convince you that if you stay reasonably close to my maintenance directions, you will never become fat again. Keep in mind that no other weight reduction program in history can boast such a large percentage of people who have kept it off after a year or more.

*19. I was told that if I drink something as innocent as one Coke I could put on five pounds. How could that be possible?*

When you reintroduce carbohydrates, you offer a dam to your body water. The weight you put on is water weight and will go away but is discouraging for a couple of days. It isn't worth it: pass it by.

*20. What about exercise?*

I don't prescribe a formal exercise program. Contrary to popular opinion, exercise does not increase your appetite. (Ask any athlete who has just won the 100-yard-dash whether he's hungry.) Moderate exercise is fine. If you increase the amount of exercise you do, you'll burn up more energy and thus hasten yourself to the success finish line. I encourage walking.

You've 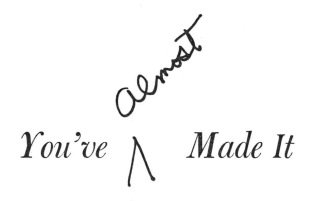 Made It

# 23

## *Refeeding*

You've done it! In many ways it's not too fanciful to say you've been reborn. Like a chick emerging from a shell of fat. After every other attempt to slim down failed, you tried the Last Chance Diet with its protein-sparing fast—and it worked! You are now slim—and ready to begin the second phase of the program.

You will be at the point where you must start eating again. Some of my patients fear that the weight is going to come back once they start eating. It doesn't.

During the refeeding period, which usually lasts from three to four weeks, you are reintroduced to eating—including carbohydrates. We want to bring your body out of ketosis, not because ketosis is an undesirable state, but because to remain in it could be like keeping you on natural diet pills for the rest of your life.

Because you are no longer in ketosis, you might start feeling a pang or two of hunger. But you must learn to adjust to a twinge of hunger now and then. That's part of life. Minor hunger must be controlled without immediately retreating to the refrigerator to satisfy it.

The important thing that must be stressed during the refeeding period is NO SALT.

Carbohydrates alone will dam up fluids. Add salt to that and a condition known as "refeeding edema" could result, meaning some added weight as measured by the scale. The weight wouldn't be fat, but still could be psychologically devastating.

The body has to have time to adapt to carbohydrates again. After all, you have been on straight protein. Once the body has that time, salt can be reintroduced to the diet.

In the meantime I strongly urge my patients to take no chances with salt. The foods selected for the refeeding diet are ones low in sodium. Follow the diet exactly. Salt can be hidden in unlikely places. A tomato, for example, has four milligrams of sodium, while a four-ounce glass of canned tomato juice has 240 milligrams.

Here is our refeeding diet. All my patients receive this standardized sheet. While the maintenance diet may be modified to fit individual needs to some extent, almost everyone follows this part exactly.

# REFEEDING DIET OF DR. LINN'S PROTEIN-SPARING FAST PROGRAM

### BREAKFAST

Tea or coffee in any quantity. Three tablespoons of skim milk may be used in a 24-hour period. Saccharin or other artificial sweeteners may be used.

### LUNCH

One selection from each of the three groups of foods listed below.

3 P.M.—PROLINN—½ ounce

### DINNER

One selection from each of the three groups of foods listed below.

8 P.M.—PROLINN—½ ounce

### FOOD SELECTIONS

*Group 1:* 4 oz. to be chosen from the following:

Veal  
Steak or hamburger  
Chicken breast  
Skim milk cottage cheese

Fresh white fish, i.e. flounder, haddock, etc.  
Tuna (in water)  
Shrimp  
One egg

*Group 2:* One type of vegetable only to be chosen from
the following (½ to ⅔ cup):

| | |
|---|---|
| Chicory | Cabbage |
| Lettuce | French style string beans |
| Onions | Broccoli |
| Turnip greens | Brussels sprouts |
| Green peppers | Cauliflower |
| Cucumbers (skinless) | Squash |
| Red Radishes | Okra |
| Tomato | Eggplant |
| Asparagus | Endive |
| Mushrooms | Escarole |

*Group 3:* D-zerta gelatin (any flavor)—one serving

## NOTE

(1) Non-caloric liquids, i.e., coffee, tea, water, diet
soda (sugarless) and seltzer. At least one quart of
liquid should be consumed daily. (DIET SODA
AND SELTZER SHOULD BE LIMITED TO 10
OZ. PER DAY)

(2) No salt may be used, but food can be made palatable by the use of a salt substitute.

(3) All canned foods should be avoided if possible.

(4) No other medication or laxative without the Doctor's knowledge.

(5) Make sure you take the nutritional supplements
you are given.

*Under no Circumstances Should Anything be Omitted
During the Course of a Day.*

ALL THINGS NOT LISTED ARE FORBIDDEN.

*THIS PHASE OF THE PROGRAM
IS EXTREMELY IMPORTANT!*

(You might notice that this is one point in the program that your intake of diet soda is limited. Sodium is the problem here. There is some sodium in low-cal soda and therefore, you must be careful about the amount you drink now.)

What we are doing here is literally reintroducing you to food. You eat from memory—a very important component in your desire for food. You remember how the strawberry shortcake tasted and you want a repeat performance. If you have never had strawberry shortcake before, it's not going to come to mind when you're thinking about eating.

It's like the infant who is introduced to one solid food at a time. If after two years, he's never tried peas, chances are he may not like them.

One aspect of the fasting period is that it dims your memory from food. Your food memory bank might not be entirely erased, but it will be blurred. So that the half a cup of string beans you will be eating now is going to seem just as desirable and tantalizing as a whole pepperoni pizza or a grand marnier souffle might have once seemed.

It is now that my patients start their regular visits

with my dietician and behavorial therapist. Their weight is down to where it should be. They have new attitudes about themselves and their bodies but at this point we start to give them new attitudes and behavior patterns toward food.

# 24

## *Putting Your Head in the Same Shape as Your Body*

*Obesity is a learned behavior disorder.
Permanent weight control requires
changes in people's habits and behavior.
Unless the patient is re-educated to
the proper way of eating, weight loss
cannot be maintained.*

—MAXENE M. KAIZEN, dietician and
behavioral therapist


Having reached this point in the program—the maintenance diet—you have reached your weight loss goal. You are no longer a fatty—at least outwardly. In your head, however, you may still be the same fat person, carrying the same baggage of bad habits that got you fat.

Habits. They are behavior formed by frequent repetition. They've become automatic so you perform them almost unconsciously. Your previous bad eating habits were things you learned and things you repeated. But what has been learned can be unlearned. Just because you've always eaten twelve times a day, sitting, standing or lying down while watching television, talking on the phone and doing a crossword puzzle, doesn't mean that you have to—or will continue to—do these things for the rest of your life. You need not be a slave to your habits.

The maintenance portion of my program is just as important as the protein-sparing fast for it is here that you are retrained. The bad habits are gradually erased and replaced with beneficial ones—habits and patterns that will put your head in the proper operating frame to keep your body as thin as it has become at the end of your fast.

What we're talking about is behavior modification, a discipline which may seem at odds with more traditional theories of psychoanalysis because, as one writer put it, "it does not take years of scratching at deep-seated psychological roots to bring about changes."

Experiments in behavior modification from Dr. John B. Watson's famous one, "The Case of Little Albert," to B.F. Skinner, have shown that almost any reaction or emotion can be learned and unlearned. Love can be transformed to hate. Fear to security. And so on. Likewise those things that you have done that had you yo-yoing up and down the scale can be altered. Just because you have been in the habit of snacking or overeating doesn't mean you can't break yourself of it.

The first thing you have to do is find out what you've been doing wrong. That entails record-keeping, strict record-keeping. Lapses in eating when you start the maintenance dict are undesirable but less important than lapses in your record-keeping.

On the next page is a chart that you should fill in daily—one page for each day.

When filling in the time you spent eating, don't approximate. If you spent four minutes eating, record four minutes and not five. If it was thirteen, it should be listed as such and not rounded off to fifteen.

Keeping track of the setting is very important. Do you eat in one place, say the kitchen, or do you eat everywhere in the house from the bathroom to the hall closet? Whenever you put anything in your mouth, this sheet should be with you. Put down the exact place you've eaten.

The physical position—standing, sitting, lying down?

Did you eat alone or did you have company?

Associated activity—now be honest, were you *just* eating or were you eating *and* doing something else like reading or watching Walter Cronkite?

Measure your degree of hunger on a scale of zero to five with zero meaning no hunger and five meaning famished.

What was your mood when you began to eat? Happy, contented, depressed, angry? Food is a sedative and is used by many people as a drug or an appeaser. When you're tense or angry do you run to the pantry for your pacifier?

And then, of course, list what you ate and how much.

Date:_____    FOOD INTAKE RECORD    Name._____

Weight: _____

| Time Start. End. | Setting | Phys. position | Alone or with Whom | Associated Activity | Degree of Hunger | Mood | Food and Amount |
|---|---|---|---|---|---|---|---|
| 6 - 11 | | | | | | | |
| 11 - 4 | | | | | | | |
| 4 - 9 | | | | | | | |
| 9 - 6 | | | | | | | |

Most people have an appalling lack of awareness about what they eat. In one study, mothers were asked about the meal patterns of their families. The answer was almost a universal, "They eat three times a day." However, after several weeks of record-keeping the mothers were astonished to find that their families subsisted mainly on snacks and junk food—every conceivable kind of candy, potato chip, cookie and the like—as long as it was packaged nicely and easy to get from the box to the mouth. Their families were having as many as twenty contacts with food a day!

After a very few days of keeping the chart, your habits that need to be broken become readily apparent.

Take the case of Joan B. who started the protein-sparing fast weighing 174¾ pounds, far too much weight for her five-foot-six and three-quarter-inch frame. Joan's reaction to the fast was similar to most of my patients, "I love it," she said, "It's so much easier to eat nothing than it is to eat a small amount."

Seven weeks later, Joan went on to the refeeding program weighing 136 pounds. In three weeks she was placed on the maintenance diet weighing just over 130.

Joan, like all my other patients, had actually started her lesson in behavior modification from the first day at my clinic. On that initial day, one of the first things she filled out was the dietician's questionnaire. Joan was asked such questions as, have you ever dieted before? Which diet? Were you successful? Meals, where eaten, when, with whom? Meals skipped, where, when, how often? Food preparation, by whom? What kind of meals do you eat away from home and in what type of restaurant? Your snacking patterns, how often, what types? Food likes and dislikes? Where you've gotten your previous information on nutrition, from advertising, magazines or books?

At that time the dietician explained to Joan that the information would be used later in modifying habits.

After the refeeding, Joan received the standard diet we give to almost all of our patients. (I will go into detail on the maintenance diet itself in the next chapter.)

After a week of filling out the sheets, Joan's major eating problem became apparent. Joan had the habit of eating all over her house, in the kitchen, living room, and bedroom.

It is very important to limit your eating to one room—preferably the kitchen—or at the most, two, the kitchen and the dining room. You associate eating with different activities and different places. If you eat in the living room, just walking into the living room can be a cue. "Wait," your mind says, "I'm in the living room. I've eaten in the living room before. I think I'll eat in the living room again." So off you go on still another pilgrimage to the kitchen for something to put in your mouth— *when you are not even hungry.*

Your job now is to erase that eating cue. If you no longer eat in the living room, the room itself will no longer act as a trigger for eating. It is a discipline, a control. But by keeping the records, you are now aware of what you must do.

The next step is to set a goal. Concentrate during the

next week on not eating in the offending room. If you are going to eat, select one spot, and do it there.

Just as the setting can act as a cue, so can an unrelated activity. Don't mix other activities with your eating. *Eating should be a pure experience.* I repeat. *Easting should be a pure experience.*

Not only does watching television or reading while you eat act as a cue to start you eating, it interferes with your knowing when to stop. Your body will tell you when your hunger—the physical property of appetite—is appeased. It sends a signal to your brain. But if your mind is occupied in watching Mary Hartman, Mary Hartman worry, worry, or in trying to figure out who "dun" it in the latest paperback mystery, it's not going to receive and act properly on the hunger signal. You will keep on eating just because you don't know you're full.

Robert D.'s doctor ordered him to try the Last Chance Diet. Robert was six-feet-one-inch, but his height in no way could handle his 302½ pounds.

"Take off at least one hundred pounds," his doctor told him.

Twelve weeks on the protein-sparing fast and Robert weighed 198 pounds. He lost another two pounds on the refeeding diet and now was all set to find out where his eating problems lie.

They lie, or more appropriately sat, right in front of the television set.

Robert loved to plop in front of the TV with a beer in one hand and a bag of pretzels in the other. He was a classic case of a "commercial food runner." As soon as the virtues of a toilet paper or a scouring powder were being extolled, Robert ran for refills in the kitchen.

As soon as his show began again, Robert would mindlessly stuff his mouth with pretzel after pretzel. There was no real pleasure involved with this eating, it was merely habit, something he always had done while watching television. Within a few weeks, Robert was able to train himself that his mouth didn't have to be full while watching "All in the Family." He could enjoy his shows just as much without eating.

Why such an emphasis on the exact number of minutes it takes you to eat? Because chances are you eat too fast. I would say more than ninety percent of my patients started out as fast eaters.

Slow down.

Enjoy your food.

Really taste it.

There are some helpful hints on slowing your eating that may seem silly at first glance, but they work and you should adhere to them.

Don't go to the table tense or keyed up. If need be, sit for a few minutes away from the table and away from the food. Get your head ready for a pleasurable, self-contained experience.

When you get to the table, don't start eating right away. Take a minute, build it up to two minutes, with the food in front of you without tasting it. *You control the food, it does not control you.* You are a thinking, reasoning human being who has control over many—if not most—of your emotions. You may get angry with someone, but you don't punch him in the nose. You may desire someone sexually, but you don't force them into sexual acts. And so you may desire to eat, but you can control what you eat and how much you eat. Your head can do it. So sit there and show yourself that you're not compulsive. Sure it's a little head game, but it will build your self esteem.

Setting a specific goal, no matter how small, and reaching it will give you more confidence in yourself and increase your pride.

Once you do start your meal, don't rush it. Take a bite. Put the fork down. Chew your food. Take one bite at a time, always putting the utensil down before taking the next bite. Stretch out the meal, give your body a chance to send that "You've had enough" signal to your brain. If you eat too fast, you'll be full and stuffed before you've had a chance to realize it.

Once the meal is over, get up, leave the table. Your eating time is for eating. It's a time for relaxation—but also concentration on the task at hand.


With all due apologies to Nedick's and other fast-food outlets, never eat while standing up. You want to be relaxed while you're eating so that you are aware of what you're consuming. Standing up is not conducive to the proper frame of mind.

One of the most dangerous places to be standing is at the refrigerator door. For some reason, many people have brain-washed themselves into believing that a bite here and a bite there while you're standing up doesn't count. Think of the cook who spends a couple of hours creating a delectable gourmet meal, but by the time it's ready to go on the table, she or he's not hungry.

"Can't understand," they'll say. "Haven't eaten all day, but I'm still not hungry."

They're not hungry because they've eaten the equivalent of a meal and a half by nibbling and tasting.

Five-foot-two Mary D. came to me weighing 143¼ pounds. In five weeks she was down to 115, where she wanted to be, but was very curious, and mildly apprehensive as to whether bad eating habits of 43 years could be changed.

Again, her problem eating area was not hard to determine. Mary was a very active and harried nurse. Her working hours ran from 7 a.m. to 3 p.m. And once she got home, she camped out in the kitchen. Her hectic day left her tired and hungry. So she would snack—right through to dinner. Her hunger, being quickly appeased was not what kept her in the kitchen. The food became her tranquilizer and also her time-consumer. She never knew quite what to do with that block of time from when she got home to when her husband arrived for dinner.

Hunger was not the key factor. Her chart showed it. For most of the snacks from three to six, the hunger box was filled with a zero. Until she kept her chart, Mary had no idea that she actually wasn't hungry.

We counseled Mary to plan in advance some activity—other than eating—to fill that time. With the new awareness of what she was doing—even though she had been doing something similar for most of her life—Mary began to be able to cope with her hangup and very soon was confining meals to times of hunger.

Sally L. didn't need anyone to tell her she needed to lose weight. At five-foot-six-inches, the 263 pounds she was carrying made that fact all too clear.

She decided to take that last chance I was offering, and she lost 113 pounds. She lost another five pounds on her four-week refeeding diet and was then in the right mind-frame to change her eating habits.

Sally had something to cope with when it came to food. She ran a small luncheonette and was constantly around food. She had been one of those people who never counted the food eaten while standing up—and Sally was always standing up and nibbling.

Sometimes she would feed guilty and spit the food out before swallowing it. My dietician had to explain that this practice was bad on two counts. One, Sally was still getting some of the calories from the food, whether she swallowed it or not. And two, she was actually teasing and tempting herself by tasting the food.

Sally had to set her mind to not nibble, to not throw that extra piece of bacon from a bacon, lettuce and tomato sandwich into her mouth instead of the refrigerator, to not lick off the peanut butter knife, to not sample the corner of the apple pie. It wasn't long before Sally had mastered the don't-eat-while-standing technique. Eating became more enjoyable to her because she now gave herself time to enjoy it.

A lot of people eat when they're depressed, tired or unhappy. Eating is not a beneficial way of overcoming these down moods. For one thing, eating to feel better won't get you feeling better, it will only get you fat.

When you find yourself heading for the kitchen when you're in a funk, change course. Get yourself to a room that isn't a cue for eating. Take a second or a minute or a few to get a grip on your feelings. Tell yourself that eating is not going to help your problem. Control yourself.

Again, the mood box on your food intake record is important. It may be one of the first times that you associate a mood with eating. Obviously you are in one kind of a mood or another when you eat—even if it's just contentment. I'm now asking you to become aware of it. You may find, that those extra jaunts to the stove coincide with certain moods. Knowing that, you can be on your guard when you find yourself feeling depressed or unhappy.

Again, the object of the record-keeping and the importance of being accurate is to make you aware of what you do. You can't possibly change something about your behavior if you don't know what your behavior is, which explains why past admonitions from doctors, friends or magazine articles to "exercise self-control and willpower" were not much use to you. These are nebulous concepts that gave you little or nothing in which to get your teeth.

Identification, first. Modification, second.

What are some of the things you should watch for and should do to change your way of eating? I recommend to my patients that they do the following, some of which might at first appear to be simplistic, but try them, they work.

Make eating a series of small steps—taking the food from the refrigerator, preparing it, putting it on the plate, etc., to give yourself more of a chance to stop the process before the food is in your stomach.

Don't buy prepared food. Work for your food. Prepare from scratch.

Eat in only one room.

Make a production out of the meal with a proper table setting.

Use the same colored dishes, napkins, and table covering.

Take smaller portions.

Serve your portions in the kitchen. Don't put serving dishes on the table.

Set your utensil down between bites.

Stop in the middle of the meal for a couple of minutes.

Make only enough for one meal. Either throw out leftovers or freeze them.

Drink water. It helps to fill you.

Never grocery shop before a meal when you're hungry. Make a list. Stick to it. Grocery shop alone so you won't be affected by another person's lack of control.

Just to show you have mastered the food, don't finish everything on your plate.

If you think you'll want two of something, like a hot dog, prepare one first. Eat it. Then prepare the second. It will give you a chance to change your mind about eating the second. Whereas, if it's already cooked, you'll be more likely to eat it—hungry or not.

Don't keep prepared munchy food in the house. What isn't there, you can't eat.

Keep foods in covered containers, out of sight.

Use smaller plates.

Increase your exercise—park a little further away from the store than you normally do. Take the stairs whenever possible. Stand when you would normally sit. Join the "Y" for some organized activity. Do more than what you've been doing.

Don't rush through your meals. Slow down.

Make eating a pure experience. Just eating, no television, newspaper, or book.

Pretty much decide what you're going to order *before* you're confronted with a restaurant's tempting menu.

You're down to where you want to be, now stay there. It can be done. *You* can do it. Just remember what your goals are and which is important—that transitory sensation in your mouth or the constant satisfaction and awareness of your thin, healthy self?

# 25

## The Maintenance Diet

THE MAINTENANCE DIET is the eating plan you should follow pretty much for the rest of your life. It's balanced and will keep you healthy.

Once you've become comfortable and sure of your new habits and control, you can ease up somewhat on strict adherence to the diet.

There will be times that you want to modify it, perhaps to include a dessert. If you do, keep the portion small and cut out the bread part of the plan that day and the next.

This is a guideline. Follow it as closely as possible.

The first month after refeeding, my patients are asked to eat the following:

## LAST CHANCE DIET REGIMEN-MAINTENANCE
### (1st Month)

### BREAKFAST

Coffee or tea in any quantity
1 small glass of tomato, grapefruit, or orange juice,
   or ½ grapefruit

### LUNCH

*Group 1* Select ¼ lb. (4 oz.) from the following:

| | |
|---|---|
| Veal | White fish (flounder, |
| Lean beef | haddock, etc. |
| Chicken | Tuna (in water) |
| 1 all-beef hot dog | Lobster |
| Skim milk cottage cheese | Crab |
| | Shrimp |

*Group 2* Select two ½ cup servings or one 1 cup
   serving of the following vegetables:

| | |
|---|---|
| Spinach | Tomato |
| Chard | Celery |
| Chicory | Dill pickle |
| Beet-greens | Asparagus |
| Lettuce | Cabbage |
| Sauerkraut | French style string beans |
| Onions | Parsley |
| Green pepper | Broccoli |
| Cucumbers | Brussels sprouts |
| Red radishes | Cauliflower |

*Group 3* Two slices of bread *daily* (may be eaten at
     at Lunch or Dinner)

*Group 4* Select one of the following:

| | |
|---|---|
| 1 apple | 1 medium peach |
| 1 orange | 2 small plums |
| ½ grapefruit | ¾ cup berries (straw., |
| 1 slice canteloupe | rasp., black.) |
| 1 slice honeydew melon | 1 pear |

### DINNER

Select one from each of the above lunch groups.

### NOTE

(1) *Beverages:* Coffee, tea, water, diet soda (sugar-
     less), and seltzer in any quantity. Saccharin or
     other artificial sweeteners may be used.

(2) *Seasonings:* Salt, pepper, vinegar, mustard,
     catsup, horseradish, onion, garlic, sweet basil,
     parsley, thyme, lemon juice, and low calorie
     salad dressing. No additional butter or fat may
     be used in preparation of food.

(3) Remember that snacks can add many extra calo-
     ries to the daily total. Budget between meal
     snacks from your daily food portions.

Success in maintaining your weight will depend
on two factors:

*YOUR DESIRE AND HOW CAREFULLY YOU
FOLLOW YOUR PROGRAM*

After the first month more food is added to the plan —we are still reintroducing you to eating. If you are someone of normal metabolism at your new low weight, this is more or less the eating plan you should stick to from now on. It is something to use as a base, though you need not be compulsive about it. You will have become aware of your eating pitfalls so that if you should start to stray, go back to following this plan more closely. But always keep it in mind.

## LAST CHANCE DIET REGIMEN-MAINTENANCE
### (2nd Month)

#### BREAKFAST

Coffee or tea in any quantity
1 small glass of tomato, grapefruit, or orange juice, or ½ grapefruit

#### LUNCH

*Group 1* Select ¼ lb. (4 oz.) from the following. All excess fat should be removed from meat. Meats and fish should be baked, boiled, or broiled.

| | |
|---|---|
| Veal | Lobster |
| Lean beef | Crab |
| Chicken | Shrimp |
| Skim milk cottage cheese | All-beef hot dog |
| 1 egg (any style) | Salmon (water packed) |
| White fish | Cold cuts (lean) |
| Tuna (in water) | |

*Group* 2  Select two ½ cup servings or one 1 cup serving
of the following:

| | |
|---|---|
| Asparagus | Lettuce |
| Broccoli | Mushrooms |
| Brussels Sprouts | Okra |
| Cabbage | Peppers |
| Cauliflower | Sauerkraut |
| Cucumber | Spinach |
| Eggplant | String beans |
| Escarole | Summer squash |
| Greens | Tomato |

*Group* 3  Two slices of bread *daily* (may be eaten at
Lunch or Dinner)

*Group* 4  Select one of the following:

| | |
|---|---|
| 1 apple | ¾ cup berries (straw., |
| 1 orange |   rasp., black.) |
| ½ cup grapefruit | 1 pear |
| 1 slice canteloupe | 10 large cherries |
| 1 slice honeydew melon | ½ cup applesauce |
| 1 medium peach | 2 medium apricots |
| 2 large plums | 2 medium dried prunes |

### DINNER

Select one from each of the above lunch groups.

### NOTE

(1) *Beverages:* same as the previous month
(2) *Seasonings:* same as the previous month

(3) Remember that snacks can add many extra calories to the daily total. Budget between meal snacks from your daily food portions.

(4) Now you may eat the following foods as often as you feel it is necessary: bouillon, broth or consomme (fat free), cranberries (without sugar), gelatin unsweetened (flavored or unflavored), low calorie salad dressing, meat sauces (without sugar), pickles, (dill or sour), rhubarb (without sugar), celery, radishes.

For people with diabetes, hypoglycemia, gout, etc., special consideration has to be given to their lifelong diets. The hypoglycemic for example, will have to eat more often—although still consuming the same amount by the end of the day. This person will generally have breakfast, a snack, lunch, a snack, dinner, and a snack.

Someone with hypertension will have to be careful of food with a lot of salt in it. Their diet will be more similar to the one during refeeding, but the quantities will be greater.

There is always the danger when presenting a standardized diet of giving the mistaken impression that everyone can be thrown into the same mold. Not so. People are individuals and have to be treated as such.

There can—and should—be some flexibility in the maintenance diet. You don't want to be too rigid otherwise you might get bored. Here are some examples of exchanges that you can make and still not worry about gaining weight.

## MAINTENANCE EXCHANGE LIST

The meats, vegetables and fruits listed on the Maintenance Diet Sheet, are very important foods that supply protein, carbohydrates, vitamins, and minerals to the diet. These foods should not be omitted from the daily food allowance. In reference to the bread group, you are permitted to consume two (2) slices of bread daily. They need not be used in this form, but can be substituted by other foods. Should there be a day, where you find yourself in a situation where you would like a cocktail or other foods not contained in the diet, the following food list deals with substitutes for the bread group:

Bread Exchange: One slice of bread =

| | |
|---|---|
| Spaghetti | ½ cup |
| Rice | ½ cup |
| Noodles | ½ cup |
| Cereals, dry | ¾ cup |
|     cooked | ½ cup |
| Bagel | ½ |
| Pancake, waffle | one medium size |
| Muffin, Biscuits | ½ |
| Potatoes, white, whole | one small |
|     white, mashed | ½ cup |
| Wine, table | 3 ounces |
| Gin, rum, vodka, & whiskey | 1 ounce |

To begin with, measure what you eat. Weigh meat before cooking and seafood after. Cook chicken with the skin on to keep the juices in, but remove the skin before eating. Mete out your portions of vegetables. After a while you will get the same practiced eye of your neighborhood butcher who scoops out hamburger to within an ounce of the weight you requested.

If you are, by chance, someone who needs an energy boost in the morning to get you going, take something from your lunch and move it to breakfast—the egg or cottage cheese, for example. Your needs may differ from someone else's. Make the maintenance diet work for you.

This is not a reducing diet. You will have already lost your weight. This is a guideline for keeping you down where you should be. You can now be the master of your eating impulses. You can recognize what little traps you fell into in the past that made you gain that hated excess weight. But now you can have the awareness of what you need to control and can make the weeks you experienced the protein-sparing fast really worthwhile—by not gaining that unwanted weight back.

The Last Chance Diet should be the last diet you'll ever need. It can be. Now it's up to you.

Enjoy the thin you, for that's what you really were all along.

# Notes on Nutrition

Emphasized throughout this book are the very real health dangers of obesity. A major motivating factor in your losing weight should have been a desire to become a healthy, good-feeling person.

So now you're there. You have your weight under control. The maintenance diet, which you will use as your framework for eating, is a sound, nutritional plan. But you will be using it as a framework, so, perhaps, a short course in nutrition and what constitutes "good" nutrition, is in order.

You will probably remember some of this from your fourth grade science lessons or in whatever grade the four food groups were explained to you.

Basically, to function efficiently, under normal non-fasting conditions, your body needs a combination of protein, carbohydrates, fats, vitamins, minerals, and water. No one food contains everything you need. One particular food will usually be a good source for one of the elements and contain only minimal amounts of the others.

Let's take a look at these various elements, their functions, and food sources.

## PROTEIN

Protein is essential for the body cells. It is needed for them to grow, to maintain them, and repair them. I've already mentioned that in the digestive process proteins are broken down into amino acids. Of these twenty-odd amino acids, eight are essential. These cannot be manufactured by the body; they must be supplied. A food will be labeled as having a "high nutritional value" when it contains a large amount of the essential amino acids.

Protein is also used by antibodies to fight infection and disease, by enzymes and hormones for the regulation of body processes and in the structure of hemoglobin—the red blood cells. PROTEIN FOOD SOURCES: Meats, fish, poultry, milk and milk products, eggs, soybeans, beans and peas, nuts, grains and cereals.

## CARBOHYDRATES

Carbohydrates consist of sugars and starches. Under nonfasting conditions, they are the body's principal source of energy. As you know too well, ingesting too many carbohydrates leads to their storage in the form of fat.

Cellulose is a complex carbohydrate which is needed —when you're not fasting—for bulk and proper elimination. CARBOHYDRATE FOOD SOURCES: cereal, bread, cakes, crackers, spaghetti and other pasta, rice, some fruits and vegetables (potatoes, sweet potatoes, bananas, lima beans, corn, dried fruits, sweetened fruits, dried legumes), syrups, jellies, jams, honey, sugars, candy, soft drinks.

## FATS

Fats are used mainly as an energy source. However they do provide protection to various internal organs, help maintain body temperature and some contain large quantities of needed vitamins.

Fat will also stave off hunger by delaying the emptying time of the stomach. FAT FOOD SOURCES: Butter, margarine, most cheeses, cream, fatty meats, shortenings, salad dressing, mayonnaise, egg yolks, peanut butter, nuts, fried foods, chocolates, rich desserts.

## MINERALS

The hard tissues of the body have minerals iln them. For instance, the bones and teeth have large amounts of calcium and potassium. But minute quantities of other minerals are needed to carry on life processes. Muscles, nerves, and the heart must be fed by body fluids containing a correct proportion of such minerals as sodium, potassium, and calcium. The approximately 15 different minerals needed by the body must be obtained from food and drink. Here is a partial list of minerals, their functions, and sources.

| MINERAL | NEEDED FOR | SOURCE |
|---|---|---|
| Calcium | bones and teeth; healthy nerves and muscle; blood clotting; healing of wounds and broken bones | milk and cheese particularly; also ice cream, shellfish, canned sardines and salmon (with bones), egg yolk, soybeans, and green vegetables |
| Copper | manufacture of hemoglobin; metabolism of iron; normal blood vessels | meats (especially liver), shellfish, dried legumes, nuts, cereal, cocoa, chocolate |
| Iodine | prevention of goiter; body energy regulation | iodized salt, seafoods |
| Iron | formation of hemoglobin; prevention of anemia | liver, heart, kidney, liver sausage, shellfish, lean meats, egg yolk, soybeans, dried beans and lentils, dried fruits, nuts, whole grain or enriched cereals and cereal products |
| Magnesium | structure of bones and teeth; transmission of nerve impulses; muscle contraction; activation of enzymes used for metabolism of carbohydrates and energy | nuts, meats, legumes, cereals |

| MINERAL | NEEDED FOR | SOURCE |
|---------|-----------|--------|
| *Phosphorus* | use with calcium for bones and teeth; for enzymes used in body metabolism; regulation of acid/base balance in body | fish, meat, poultry, milk, cheeses, whole grain cereals, legumes, nuts |
| *Potassium* | synthesis of proteins; fluid balance maintenance; healthy nerves and muscles; enzyme reactions | fish, meat, cereals, fruits, vegetables |
| *Sodium* | fluid balance maintenance; acid/base balance in body; absorption of other nutrients including glucose | table salt, fish, meat, poultry, eggs, milk, foods where salt used as preservative |
| *Zinc* | wound healing; normal growth and development | green leafy foods, fruits, whole grains, organ meats, lean meats |

## VITAMINS

Vitamins are essential for food to be used properly and for the body to function properly. The functions of vitamins vary with the particular vitamin. Vitamin A, for example, is needed for healthy skin, mucus membranes, and night vision. Vitamin K is essential for normal blood-clotting. Deficiencies over an extended time period can lead to a variety of symptoms including night blindness and skin lesions or actual deficiency diseases such as rickets and scurvy.

There are two types of vitamins, fat soluble and water soluble.

Fat soluble, which include A, D, E, and K are not needed daily in your diet. If you take in more than you need of this type of vitamin, the excess will be stored by your body. A deficiency of a fat soluble vitamin is slow to develop.

Water soluble vitamins (Vitamin C, the B Vitamins) must be supplied daily, any excess is excreted in the urine with only minimal storage. Deficiency symptoms of this type of vitamin may develop rapidly.

Here then are some of the vitamins, their uses and sources.

| VITAMIN | NEEDED FOR | SOURCE |
| --- | --- | --- |
| *Vitamin A* | healthy skin, bones, and teeth; growth; resistance of infection; good vision | liver, egg yolk, deep yellow and dark green leafy vegetables, tomatoes, liver sausage, butter, margarine, cheese made from whole milk |
| *Vitamin D* | absorption and utilization of calcium and phosphorus; healthy bones; strong teeth | liver, egg yolk, liver sausage, foods fortified with Vitamin D such as "Vitamin D Milk" and evaporated milk, exposure to direct sunlight |
| *Vitamin B₁ (Thiamine)* | using carbohydrates for energy; healthy nervous system | pork, organ meats such as liver, heart, and kidney; whole grain and enriched breads and cereals, peas and beans, nuts, eggs |

| VITAMIN | NEEDED FOR | SOURCE |
|---|---|---|
| *Vitamin B2* *(Riboflavin)* | using protein, fats, and carbohydrates for energy and tissue building; healthy skin (in particular around mouth, nose, and eyes) | organ meats like liver, heart, kidney, and tongue, liver sausage, milk, cheese, eggs, meats, green leafy vegetables, enriched breads and cereals, dried beans |
| *Niacin* | healthy nervous system and skin; normal digestion; helping cells to use oxygen to release energy | liver, meats, fish, whole grain or enriched breads and cereals, dried peas and beans, nuts, peanut butter |
| *Vitamin B6* *(Pyridoxine)* | protein utilization; normal growth; prevention of certain types of anemia; normal utilization of copper and iron | organ meats such as liver and kidney, meats and fish, whole grain cereals, soybeans, tomatoes, peanuts and peanut butter, corn |
| *Pantothenic Acid* | breakdown of carbohydrates, fats, and proteins for energy production; synthesis of fatty acids, sterols, and steroid hormones, and amino acids | organ meats, egg yolk, meats and fish, soybeans, peanuts and peanut butter, broccoli, cauliflower, sweet potatoes, peas, cabbage, potatoes, whole grain products |
| *Folic Acid* | development of red blood cells; normal metabolism of carbohydrates, proteins, and fats | organ meats such as liver and kidney, asparagus, turnips, spinach, kale, broccoli, corn, cabbage, lettuce, potatoes, nuts |

| VITAMIN | NEEDED FOR | SOURCE |
|---|---|---|
| Vitamin B12 | red blood cell production in bone marrow; building new protein; normal functioning of nervous tissue | liver and kidney, lean meats and fish, oysters, hard cheeses, milk |
| Vitamin C (Ascorbic Acid) | building the "cement" that holds cells together; healthy teeth, gums, and blood vessels; improving iron absorption; resisting infections and aiding wound healing; syntheziation of hormones to regulate body functions | citrus fruits (oranges, grapefruit, lemons), strawberries, cantaloupes, raw or slightly cooked vegetables—specially green peppers, cauliflower, broccoli, kale, brussels sprouts, cabbage, tomatoes, potatoes |
| Vitamin E | retardation of destruction of Vitamin A, ascorbic acid, and polyunsaturated fatty acids; protection of red blood cells | wheat germ oil, rice germ oil, cottonseed oil, green leafy vegetables, legumes, nuts, salad oils, margarines, shortenings |
| Vitamin K | normal promotion of normal blood clotting | spinach, kale, cabbage, cauliflower, pork liver |

Of course, a good multivitamin is invaluable in providing necessary vitamins and minerals that might be lacking from your diet.

Another way to divide up food is by the four food groups—milk, vegetable-fruit, meat, and bread-cereal.

Thought of in this way, you should remember that milk items are the primary sources of calcium, riboflavin, phosphorus and high quality protein. They also provide Vitamin A and D when fortified.

Vegetables and fruit contain Vitamin C along with A, some iron and other minerals.

Meat is the supplier of protein, thiamine, riboflavin, iron and niacin, while the bread group has iron, carbohydrate, and some protein.

# Bibliography

Allen, F. M.; Stillman, E. and Fritz, R.: Total Dietary Regulation in the Treatment of Diabetes. MONOGRAPH II NEW YORK, ROCKEFELLER INSTITUTE OF MEDICAL RESEARCH, 1919, p. 9097.

Aoki, T. T.; Muller, W. A.; Brennan, F. and Cahill, G. F.: Metabolic Effects of Glucose in Brief and Prolonged Fasted Man; AM. J. CLIN. NUT., 28 (5):507, 1975.

Baird, I. M., Parsons, R. L. and Howard, A. N.: Clinical and Metabolic Studies of Chemically Defined Diets in the Management of Obesity; METABOLISM, 23:645-57, 1974.

Benoit, F. L., Martin, R. L., Whatten, R. H.: Changes in Body Composition During Weight Reduction in Obesity: ANN. INTERN. MED. 63, 604, 1965.

Bistrian, B. R.; Blackburn, G. L.; Flatt, J. P.; Winterer, J.; Cochran, D. and Young, V.: Protein Requirements for Net Anabolism with a Hypocaloric Diet; CLIN RES., 23:315A, 1975.

Bistrian, B. R., Blackburn, G. L.; Flatt, J. P., Sizer, J., Scrimshaw, N. S.; Sherman, M.: Nitrogen Metabolism and Insulin

Requirement in Obese, Diabetic Adults fed a Protein Sparing Modified Fast; CLIN. RES., 23:589A, 1975.

Bistrian, B. R., Blackburn, G. L. and Scrimshaw, N. S.: Effect of Mild Infectious Illness on Nitrogen Metabolism in Patients on a Modified Fast; AM. J. CLIN. NUT., 28 (9):1044-51, 1975.

Bjurulf, P. Atherosclerosis and Body Build. with Special Reference to Size and Number of Subcutaneous Fat Cells: ACTA MED. SCAND. 166, 349, 1959.

Blackburn, G. L.; Bistrian, B. R.; Flatt, J. P.: Preservation of the Physiological Responses in a Protein-Sparing Modified Fast; CLIN. RES., 22:461A, 1974.

Blackburn, G. L., Bistrian, B. R., Flatt, J. P., Page, G. and Stone, M.: Restoration of the Visceral Component of Protein Malnutrition Using Hypocaloric Feeding; CLIN. RES., 23:315A, 1975.

Blackburn, G. L., Bistrian, B. R., Flatt, J. P. and Sizer, J.: Role of a Protein Sparing Modified Fast in a Comprehensive Weight Redouction in Recent Advances in Obesity Research: Alan Howard (Ed.), Newman Publishing, Ltd., 1975.

Blackburn, G. L., and Flatt, J. Metabolic Response to Illness; Protein-Sparing Therapy: ALIMENTARY DISORDERS 23-29, 1974.

Blackburn, G. L., and Flatt, J. Preservation of Lean Body Mass During Acute Weight Reduction: FEDERATION PROCEEDINGS 32 916, 1973.

Blackburn, G. L., and Flatt, J. The Metabolic Fuel Regulatory System; Implications for Protein-Sparing Therapies during

Blackburn, G. L.; Flatt, J. P.: Metabolic Response to Illness: Protein-Sparing Therapy: COMP. THER., 1 (5):23-29, 1975. Caloric Deprivation and Disease: AMERICAN JOURNAL CLINICAL NUTRITION 27, 175-187, February 1974.

Bloom, W. L. Inhibition of Salt Excretion by Carbohydrate: ARCH. OF INT. MED. 109, 26-32, 1962.

Bray, G., and Jordan, H. A. Sims, E. A.: Evaluation of the Obese Patient: JAMA 235, 1487-91, April 5, 1976.

Bray, G. A. The Myth of Diet in the Management of Obesity: AMER. JOURNAL CLINICAL NUTRITION: 23, 1141-1148, Sept. 1970.

Cahill, Geo. and Aoki, T. How Metabolism Afiects Clinical Problems; MEDICAL TIMES, 106-122, October, 1970.

Cahill, Geo. Starvation in Man; NEW ENGLAND MEDICAL JOURNAL, 668-675, March, 1970.

Cahill, G. F., Owen, O. E., Morgan, A.P. The Consumption of Fuels During Prolonged Starvation; ADVANCES IN ENZYME REGULATION; 6, 143-50, 1967.

Cahill, G. F., Jr.: Commentaries in "Obesities in Perspective" in *Fogarty International Series*. George Bray (Ed). H.E.W. Publisher, 1975.

Calloway, D. H., Margen, S. Variation in Endogenous Nitrogen Excretion and Dietary Nitrogen Utilization as Determinants of Human Protein Requirement; AM. JOURN. OF CLINICAL NUT., 101, 205-216, 1971.

Cutler, P., Fuller, D., Young, E., et. al. The Endless Fight Against Fat; CURRENT PRESCRIBING, 3 P. 49-60, March 1976.

Danowski, T. S. Hypoglycemia: OBESITY/BARIATRIC MEDICINE, 2, 7-11, 1973.

Danowski, T. S. The Management of Obesity: HOSPITAL PRACTICE, 39-46, April 1976.

Dorenick, E. J., Swendseid, M. E., Bland, W. H., et. al. Prolonged Starvation as Treatment for Severe Obesity: JAMA, 187, 100-105, Jan. 4, 1964.

Dorfman, S. H. and Madad, A. Floch. Low Fiber Content of Connecticut Diets: AM. JOURN. OF CLINICAL NUTRITION, 29, 87-89, Jan. 1976.

Drenick, E. J. JAMA, 1964, Vol. 187, Page 100.

Drenick, E. J., Bland, W. H., Singer, F. R.: Body Potassium Content in Obese Subjects and Potassium Depletion During Prolonged Fasting: AM. JOURNAL OF CLINICAL NUTRITION, 18, 278-85, 1966.

Drenick, E. J. Weight Reduction By Prolonged Fasting: MEDICAL TIMES, 100, 209-30, 1972.

Editorial*: Obesity—A Continuing Enigma: JAMA, 211/3, 492-493, Jan. 1970.

* Ref: Bloom, W. L. Fasting as an Introduction to the Treatment of Obesity: METABOLISM, Vol. 8, 214-220, 1959. Ball, M. F., Canary, J. J., Kyle, L. H. Tissue Changes During Intermittent Starvation and Caloric Restriction as Treat. for Severe Obesity: ARCHIVE OF OBESITY INT. MED., Vol. 125, 62-28, 1970.

El-Khodary, A. Z., Ball, M. F., Oweiss, M., et al. Insulin Secretion and Body Composition in Obesity: METABOLISM, 21, 641, 1972.

Fitzpatrick, G. F.; Mequid, M. N.; O'Connell, R. C., et. al.: Nitrogen Sparing by Carbohydrate in Man: Intermittent or Continuous Enteral Compared with Continuous Parenteral Glucose; SURG., 78 (1):105-13, 1975.

Flatt, J. P.; Blackburn, G. L.: Role of the Increased Adipose Tissue Mass in the Apparent Insulin Insensitivity of Obesity in *Recent Advances in Obesity Research:* Alan Howard (Ed), Newman Publishing, Ltd., 1975.

Freeman, J. B.; Stegnik, L. D., et al.: Evaluation of Amino Acid Infusion as Protein-Sparing Agents in Normal Adult Subjects; AM. J. CLIN. NUT. 28 (5):477-81, 1975.

Garrow, J. S. Energy Balance and Obesity in Man: NORTH-HOLLAND PUB. CO.; 1974.

Genuth, S. M.; Castro, J. A. and Vertes, V.: Weight Reduction in Obesity by Outpatient Semi-Starvation; JAMA, 230:987-91, 1974.

Genuth, S. M. and Vertes, V.: Weight Reduction by Supplemented Fasting in *Recent Advances in Obesity Research:* I. Alan Howard (Ed.), Newman Publishing, Ltd., 1975.

Grey, N.; Kipnis, D. M. Effect of Diet Composition on the Hyperinsulenemia of Obesity: NEW ENGLAND JOUR. MED., 285, 827-831, Oct. 1971.

Gordon, E. S., Goldberg, M., Chosy, G. J. A New Concept in the Treatment of Obesity: JAMA, 156-166, Oct. 1963.

Hartmann, G. "O Calorie Diet" in Obesity: PRAXIS (Medical Univ. Glin, Basel) 59/12, 431-432, 1970.

Heaton, K. W. Fiber, Blood Lipids and Heart Disease: AM. JOURNAL OF CLINICAL NUTRITION, 29, 125-126, Feb. 1976.

Hill, M. J. Colon Cancer: A Disease of Fibre Depletion or of Dietary Excess: DIGESTION, 11, 289-306, 1974.

Howard, A. N. and Baird, I. M.: The Treatment of Obesity by Low Calorie Semi-synthetic Diets in *Recent Advances in Obesity Research:* I. Alan Howard (Ed.), Newman Publishing Ltd., 1975

Huang, P. C., Young, U. R., Cholakos, B., et. al. Determination of the Minimum Dietary Essential Amino Acid-to-Total Nitrogen Ratio for Beef Protein Fed to Young Men: AMER. JOURNAL OF CLINICAL NUTRITION, 90, 416-22, 1966.

Jordan, H. A., and Levitz, L. A Behavioral Approach to the Problem of Obesity: OBESITY—PATHOGENISIS & MANAGEMENT, 155-172, Publishing Sciences Group, Inc. Press.

Jordan, H. A., and Levitz, L. A Behavioral Approach to the Problem of Obesity: OBESITY/BARIATRIC MED., 4, 58-67, 1975.

Jordan, H. A., Kimbrell, G. M., Levitz, L. Managing Obesity, Why Diet is Not Enough: POST GRADUATE MEDICINE, 59, 183-186, April 1976.

Jordan, H. A. and Levitz, L. S. Behavior Modification in a Self-Help Group: J. AM. DIET ASSOC., 62, 27-29, 1973.

Jourdan, M. H., and Bradfield, R. B. Body Composition Changes During Weight Loss Estimated from Energy, Nitrogen, Sodium and Potassium Balances: AM. JOURNAL CLIN. NUTRITION, 26, 144-149, February 1973.

Jourdan, M.; Margen, S. and Bradfield, R. B.: Protein-Sparing Effect in Obese Women Fed Low Calorie Diets; AM. J. CLIN. NUT., 27:3-12, 1974.

Kalkhoff, R. K., Kim. H. J., Cerletty, J., et. al. Metabolic Effects of Weight Loss in Obese Subjects. Changes in Plasma Substrate Levels, Insulin and Growth Hormone Responses: DIABETES, 20, 83-91, 1971.

Kjelberg, J., and Reizenstein, P. Effect of Starvation on Body Composition in Obesity: ACTA MED. SCAND., 188, 171-178, 1970.

Kolanowski, J., Pizzarro, M. A., DeGasparo, M., et al. Influence of Fasting on Adreocortical and Pancreatic Islet Response to Glucose Loads in the Obese: EUROP. JOURN. CLIN. INVEST. (Berl), 1/1, 25-31, 1970.

Kreisberg, R. A., Boshell, B. R., DiPacido, J., et al. Insulin Secretion in Obesity: NEW ENGLAND JOURN. OF MED., 276, 314-319, Feb. 1967.

Lawlor, T., and Wells, D. G. Metabolic Hazards of Fasting: AMERICAN JOUR. OF CLINICAL NUTRITION, 22 P. 1142-49, 1969.

Marliss, E. B., and Nakhooda, A. F. Ketosis and Protein-Sparing in Man: CLIN. RES., 22, 751A, 1974.

Marti-Ibañez. Personality and Obesity: MD, 13-15, March 1976.

Motil, K. J. and Pencharz, P. B.: Effectiveness and Safety of Protein-Sparing Modified Fast in Weight Reduction in Obese Adolescents; FED. PRO. 35:656, 1976.

Obesity and Diabetes: AUSTRALIAN ANNALS OF MEDICINE, Vol. 10, 1-3, Feb. 1969.

Owen, O. E., Morgan, A. P., Kemp, H. G., Cahill, G. F.: Brain Metabolism During Fasting: JOUR. CLINICAL INVESTIGATION, 46, 1589-1595, 1967.

Palm, J. Daniel, Diet Away Your Stress, Tension, & Anxiety: DOUBLEDAY 1976.

Rooth, G. Carstrom. Therapeutic Fasting: ACTA MED. SCAND., 187, 455-463, 1970.

Runcie, J., and Thomson, J. J. Prolonged Starvation—A Dangerous Procedure?; BRITISH MED. JOUR., 3, 432-435, 1970.

Scriver, C., and Rosenberg, L. Amino Acid Metabolism and Its Disorders: SAUNDERS PRESS, 1973.

Spencer, H., Lewin, I., Samachson, J. Changes in Metabolism in Obese Persons During Starvation: AMER. JOURN. OF MED., 40, P. 27-37, 1966.

Speroff, Leon. The Problem of Obesity: CONTEMPORARY OB/GYN., 5, 85-90, March 1975.

Stock, A. L., and Yudkin, J. Nutrient Intake of Subjects on Low Carbohydrate Diet Used in Treatment of Obesity: AM. JOURN. CLIN. NUTRITION, 23/7, 948-952, 1970.

Stuart, R. B. Behavioral Control of Overeating: BEHAV. RES. THER., 5, 357-365, 1967.

Stuart, R. B., and Davis, B. Slim Chance in a Fat World. Behavioral Control of Obesity: RESEARCH PRESS, 1972.

Stunkard, A. J., and Levitz, L. S. A Therapeutic Coalition for Obesity. Behavior Modification and Patient Self-help: AMER. JOURN. PSYCHIATRY, 131, 423-427, April 1974.

Swanson, D., and Dinello, F. Follow-up of Patients Starved for Obesity: PSYCHOSOMATIC MEDICINE, 32, p. 209-14, 1970.

Van Itallie, T. B., Yang, N., and Haskim, S. A.: Dietary approaches to obesity, *Metabolic and Appetitive Consideration in Recent Advances in Obesity Research:* I. Alan Howard (Ed), Nedman Publishing, Ltd., 1975.

Verdy, M. BSP Retention During Total Fasting: METABOLISM-CLINICAL AND EXPERIMENTAL, 13, p. 169, 1966.

Vinnick, L., and Peterson, R. E. Restructuring the Obese: DRUG THERAPY, 111-120, Oct. 1975.

Wauters, J. P., Busset, R. Dayer, A., Favre, H. Effects of Various Slimming Regimes on Body Composition in Simple Obesity: SCHWEIZ ED. WSCHR., 100/28, (1272-1278), Graphs 6, Tables 3, 1970.

Weisner, R. L. Fasting—A Review with Emphasis on the Electrolytes: THE AMERICAN JOURN. OF MED., 50, P. 233-40, 1971.

Weisswange, A.; Cuendet, G. S. and Marliss, F. B.: Metabolic Response to a "Revolutionary Diet." CLIN. RES. 22:482A, 1974.

Winterer, J. C.; Bistrian, B. R., Blackburn, G. L.; Young, V. R.: Effects of a Protein-Sparing Diet and Brief Fast on Total Body Protein Turnover in Obese Subjects; CLIN. RES., 23:595A, 1975.

Yalow, R. S., Glick, S. M., Roth, J., et al. Plasma Insulin and Growth Hormone Levels in Obesity and Diabetes: ANN. N. Y. ACAD. SCI., 131, 357-373, 1965.